DISCLAIMER

This book is provided for educational purposes only and is not intended as a substitute for professional medical advice, diagnosis, or treatment. While it aims to enhance communication with Spanish-speaking patients, healthcare practitioners should not solely rely on its content for making clinical decisions. The medical information within this book is a supplementary tool and does not replace the expertise of a qualified healthcare provider or the necessity of a trained medical interpreter, which may be legally required in certain contexts. Users are encouraged to always seek the advice of their medical training and judgment in clinical settings. Dependence on any information from this book is at the user's own risk. It is the responsibility of the healthcare provider to evaluate the accuracy, completeness, and usefulness of any information, opinion, advice, or other content available through this book.

TABLE OF CONTENTS

INTRODUCTION

Welcome to 'Learn Beginner Medical Spanish with Real Life Dialogues in 30 Days'!

This isn't just a book; it's your golden ticket to connecting deeply with Spanish-speaking patients.

Designed for a diverse range of healthcare professionals, this book is the perfect resource whether you are an EMT, nurse, doctor, dentist, medical assistant, physician, physician assistant, nurse practitioner, lab technician, or part of the ancillary medical staff. No matter your role in the healthcare industry, this book is tailored for you!

We've broken down your learning into 30 fun-filled days, each one a step towards celebrating your progress and making your dive into medical Spanish both thrilling and fruitful.

Picture this: You, a healthcare professional, step into a patient's room and, for the first time, comfortably converse in Spanish, bridging the gap between languages and hearts. That could be you in just 30 days.

As you embark on this journey, you'll gain practical skills for various medical scenarios. Learn to conduct patient interviews, perform examinations, and handle emergencies with confidence and empathy. Each day of this journey is crafted to be fun, engaging, and, above all, fruitful in making your dive into medical Spanish rewarding.

As you progress through each day, imagine the smiles and nods of understanding from your Spanish-speaking patients as you communicate with them.

From the first 'hola' to more complex medical consultations, each chapter in this book is a stepping stone towards confident communication. Our book also includes a comprehensive phonetic guide and a curated list of must-know medical words and phrases, designed to get you conversational quickly in real-life medical settings. Whether it's emergency scenarios or routine check-ups, you'll learn to handle a variety of situations with ease and empathy.

But that's not all. We're not just tackling language here. We're delving into the rich cultural fabric of Spanish-speaking communities. Because let's face it, mastering healthcare communication is about so much more than words. From friendly hellos to intricate medical discussions, each chapter is your secret weapon for confidently handling any medical situation.

Embrace this 30-day adventure as a transformational journey. You're not just learning Spanish; you're evolving as a healthcare provider. You're about to enhance your patient care and make meaningful connections, all while gaining a newfound respect for your Spanish-speaking patients' experiences.

Let's transform, connect, and grow together. ¡Vamos! Let's get started!

RESOURCES

FACEBOOK GROUP

- Learn Spanish - Touri Language Learning
- Learn French - Touri Language Learning

YOUTUBE

- Touri Language Learning Channel

FREE GIFTS

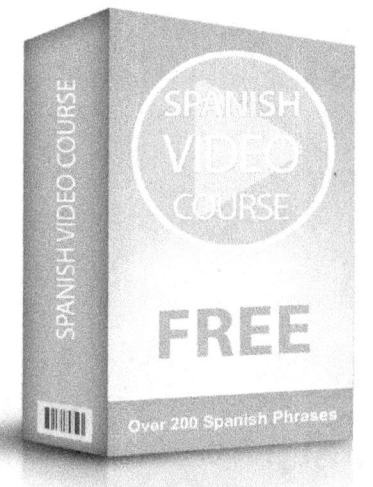

Mini Spanish Course
200+ words and phrases in audio you can start using today!

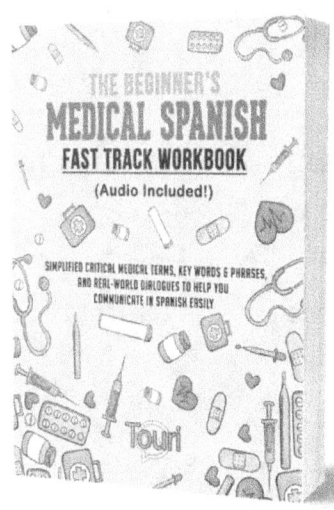

The Beginner's Medical Spanish Fast Track Workbook
Simplified Critical Medical Terms, Key Words & Phrases, and Real-World Dialogues to Help You Communicate in Spanish Easily

Get all these amazing bonuses by going to:

SCAN ME

https://bit.ly/42K1CTv

MAXIMIZING LEARNING WITH THIS BOOK

We want you to get the most out of this book, so we've put together some best practices for you. These tips will help make your learning experience both enjoyable and fruitful.

Sequential Learning
Start by reading each chapter to get familiar with the content, then revisit the same section for reinforcement. Pay special attention to pronunciation guides and contextual examples.

Interactive Exercises
Engage with the exercises provided in the book, such as translating sentences or completing dialogues, to apply what you've learned.

Writing Exercises
The book includes spaces for you to write out Spanish words or phrases, helping reinforce your learning.

Consistent Practice
Regularly revisit different sections of the book to strengthen both reading comprehension and vocabulary retention.

Dialogue Practice
Follow along with dialogues to better understand conversation structure and context.

Cultural Notes and Insights
Refer to cultural insights provided in the book to enhance your understanding of Spanish-speaking communities.

Self-Assessment
Utilize the quizzes and the recaps provided after key sections to evaluate your comprehension and progress.

Remember, the journey of learning medical Spanish is as rewarding as it is essential. By following these best practices, you'll be on your way to effectively communicating with your Spanish-speaking patients. We're excited for you to start this journey and see the incredible impact it will have on your professional life and the lives of your patients.

SPANISH FUNDAMENTALS

Welcome to "Day 1: Spanish Fundamentals," where we lay the groundwork for your medical Spanish proficiency. We start with the basics: the Spanish alphabet's distinct sounds, practical numbers for everyday use, and essential colors. You'll discover a strategic approach to rapidly build your vocabulary, key grammar essentials for structuring your sentences, and focused pronunciation practice to ensure clarity in your communication. By the end of this section, you'll be equipped with the fundamental tools for constructing basic Spanish sentences, essential for effective interactions in a healthcare setting.

The Spanish Alphabet

A	ah		**N**	en-nay
B	bay		**Ñ**	eh-nyay
C	say		**O**	oh
CH	cheh		**P**	pay
D	day		**Q**	coo
E	eh		**R**	eh-ray
F	eh-fay		**RR**	eh-rray
G	heh		**S**	eh-say
H	ah-chay		**T**	tay
I	ee		**U**	oo
J	ho-tah		**V**	bay-chee-kah
K	kah		**W**	bay-doh-blay
L	ehl-lay		**X**	eh-keys
LL	eh-yay		**Y**	ee-gree-ay-guh
M	eh-may		**Z**	zay-tah

Vowels

Spanish vowels are pure sounds unlike English vowels which vary widely. There are five vowel types, each with short and long forms as well as long forms created by diphthongs. Proper vowel pronunciation is key for understanding.

Spanish vowels each have a pure sound:

Short Vowels

- A - casa (house)
- E - eso (that)
- I - fin (end)
- O - son (they are)
- U - luz (light)

Long Vowels

- Á - máximo (maximum)
- É - bebé (baby)
- Í - país (country)
- Ó - sólo (only)
- Ú - menú (menu)

Consonants

Many Spanish consonants sound similar to English counterparts. However, there are important differences in how letters like r, h, ll or c are produced. Common problem sounds for English speakers will be highlighted.

Certain letters trip up English speakers:

- H - hablar (to speak) - always silent
- Ll - llave (key) - pronounced "y"
- Ñ - niño (child) - «ny» sound

Stress and Rhythm

Spanish is considered a syllable-timed language, structured around a rhythm of evenly spaced syllables. Words will have one main stressed syllable. Listening practice will build an ear for Spanish rhythmic flow.

Syllables sound evenly spaced. Stress falls on the second-to-last syllable:

- EnferMEra (nurse)
- PaCIENte (patient)

Numbers

Zero	**Cero**	Twenty	**Veinte**
One	**Uno**	Thirty	**Treinta**
Two	**Dos**	Forty	**Cuarenta**
Three	**Tres**	Fifty	**Cincuenta**
Four	**Cuatro**	Sixty	**Sesenta**
Five	**Cinco**	Seventy	**Setenta**
Six	**Seis**	Eighty	**Ochenta**
Seven	**Siete**	Ninety	**Noventa**
Eight	**Ocho**	One hundred	**Cien**
Nine	**Nueve**	Five hundred	**Quinientos**
Ten	**Diez**	One thousand	**Mil**

Colors

Red	**Rojo**	White	**Blanco**
Blue	**Azul**	Purple	**Morado**
Green	**Verde**	Orange	**Naranja**
Yellow	**Amarillo**	Pink	**Rosa**
Black	**Negro**	Brown	**Marrón**

How to Learn 1000 Spanish Words Instantly

Did you know that many English words have close relatives in Spanish, thanks to their common Latin roots?

It's like having a secret key to unlock a whole new set of vocabulary with minimal effort! Let's explore this fascinating linguistic connection.

Take words in English that end with 'I-O-N,' such as 'region.' In Spanish, these words often have a counterpart that is strikingly similar.

- All you need to do is add an accent on the 'o,' and voilà – 'region' becomes 'región.'

But that's not all. When you come across English words ending in 'T-I-O-N,' like 'operation,' there's a simple switch to make.

- Replace the 'T' with a 'C,' and there you have it – 'operation' transforms into 'operación' in Spanish.

These patterns reveal how closely intertwined English and Spanish are, making learning new words easier and more intuitive. Next time you encounter an English word with these endings, try applying this rule and see how quickly you can expand your Spanish vocabulary!

Grammar Essentials

Grammar provides the organizational framework for communicating. Spanish structure differs from English in word order, gendered nouns, formal/informal forms, verb conjugations and more. This section will break down the grammar vital for medical conversations.

Nouns, Articles and Adjectives

Nouns have a gender of either masculine or feminine which requires matching adjective agreement. Definite and indefinite articles also reflect this gender. Using proper nouns and descriptors is vital.

- El doctor (male doctor)
- La doctora (female doctor)

Articles precede nouns and match their gender:

- <u>La</u> sala (the room)
- <u>El</u> hospital (the hospital)

Subject Pronouns

Spanish has distinct pronoun forms for different subject perspectives (I, you, we, etc). There is also a more formal 2nd person pronoun "usted" used for polite address. Choosing the appropriate subject viewpoint shapes meaning.

Verbs

Verbs are the "action words" that drive sentences and convey key information about the patient. In Spanish, verbs conjugate based on subject perspective and change in complex ways based on tense (when the action occurs). Mastering verb flexibility is essential.

Stem-changing verbs alter vowels:
Pensar (to think) → pienso (I think)

Reflexive verbs reflect back:
Llamarse (to call oneself) → me llamo (I call myself)

Verb Tense Example

1. **Present Tense (El Presente):** Used to describe current conditions or routines.

   - "Tengo dolor" (I have pain)
   - "El paciente necesita medicamento" (The patient needs medication)

2. **Past Tense (El Pasado):** Important for discussing medical history or past symptoms.

   - Simple Past (El Pretérito): "Tuve fiebre ayer" (I had a fever yesterday)
   - Imperfect (El Imperfecto): "Tosía frecuentemente" (I used to cough frequently)

3. **Future Tense (El Futuro):** Used for discussing future appointments or treatment plans.

   - "Tendrá que hacerse una prueba" (You will have to have a test done)

Prepositions

Prepositions link nouns and give basic contextual meaning regarding direction, location and time. They commonly combine with verbs as well. Fluently using appropriate prepositions allows for clear medical communication.

1. **"En" (In/On):** Used to describe location.

   ◢ "El paciente está en la sala de espera". (The patient is in the waiting room.)

2. **"Con" (With):** Describes accompaniment or inclusion.

   ◢ "El doctor viene con los resultados". (The doctor comes with the results.)

3. **"Desde" (From):** Indicates the starting point in time or space.

   ◢ "Descansar desde las diez". (Rest from ten o'clock.)

4. **"Hasta" (Until):** Used to indicate duration.

   ◢ "Debe tomar el medicamento hasta el viernes". (You should take the medication until Friday.)

5. **"Por" (For):** Indicates the reason or motive.

   ◢ "Está aquí por una cita". (He is here for an appointment.)

6. **"A" / "Al" (To):**

   ◢ "Voy al hospital". (I go to the hospital.)

Understanding these prepositions and their correct usage is crucial for clear and effective medical communication in Spanish.

Pronunciation Practice

In learning medical Spanish, getting pronunciation right is like setting the foundation for your language skills. Think of it as building a house. If the base isn't strong, the house won't stand. That's why we focus on pronunciation first. It's crucial for making sure you're understood and can understand others. We'll start here, with the basics, to build your confidence. Then, as you get better, you'll be ready for more complex conversations and dialogues. This is your first step towards mastering medical Spanish!

Vowel Emphasis Drills

1. **"Análisis" (ah-nah-lee-sees)** - Analysis

    ◢ <u>Practice</u>: Repeat "análisis" focusing on the clear 'a' sound.
    ◢ **Exercise:** Say "El análisis de sangre" (The blood analysis) three times.

2. **"Enfermero" (en-fer-meh-roh)** - Nurse

    ◢ <u>Practice</u>: Emphasize the 'e' in "enfermero".
    ◢ **Exercise:** Say "El enfermero revisa" (The nurse checks) multiple times.

3. **"Infección" (een-fek-see-ohn)** - Infection

    ◢ <u>Practice</u>: Focus on the 'i' in "infección".
    ◢ **Exercise:** Repeat "Tiene una infección" (You have an infection).

4. **"Oído" (oh-ee-doh)** - Ear

    ◢ <u>Practice</u>: Pronounce "oído," emphasizing the 'o.'
    ◢ **Exercise:** Say "El oído del paciente" (The patient's ear) clearly.

5. **Urgencia" (oorh-hen-see-ah)** - Emergency

    ◢ <u>Practice</u>: Highlight the 'u' in "urgencia".
    ◢ **Exercise:** Repeat "Es una urgencia" (It's an emergency) several times.

Through these drills, focus on the distinct sounds of each vowel in the context of medical terms. Practice each word and sentence until the vowel sounds are clear and consistent.

Consonant Clarity

1. **"Radiografía" (rah-dee-oh-grah-fee-ah)** - X-ray

    ◢ Focus on the rolling 'r' and the hard 'g.'
    ◢ **Exercise:** Say "Usted necesita una radiografía del pecho" (You need a chest X-ray) three times.

2. **"Jarabe" (hah-rah-beh)** - Syrup

    ◢ Practice the soft 'j' sound, similar to the English 'h.'
    ◢ **Exercise:** Repeat "El jarabe para la tos" (The cough syrup) multiple times.

3. **"Llave" (yah-veh)** - Key (not a medical term, but good for the 'll' sound)

   ◢ Focus on the 'll' pronounced as 'y.'

   ◢ **Exercise:** Say "¿Dónde está la llave?" (Where is the key?) to practice the sound.

4. **"Cirugía" (seer-roo-hee-ah)** - Surgery

   ◢ Emphasize the soft 'c' which sounds like 's.'

   ◢ **Exercise:** Repeat "La cirugía fue exitosa" (The surgery was successful).

5. **"Hospital" (os-pee-tahl)** - Hospital

   ◢ Notice the silent 'h' at the beginning.

   ◢ **Exercise:** Say "Voy al hospital" (I am going to the hospital) several times.

These exercises are designed to help you practice the pronunciation of some of the trickier consonants in Spanish, essential for clear communication in a medical setting.

Basic Sentence Structures

In this section we'll go over the fundamental techniques for creating compound and complex sentences, specifically tailored for medical settings. Understanding and applying these sentence structures are crucial for effective communication in healthcare environments.

1. Building Compound Sentences

Similar to English we can combine simple sentences using conjunctions such as **'y'** (and), **'pero'** (but), and **'o'** (or).

Example:

⊿ **Simple Sentence 1:**

- "El paciente tiene fiebre".
  (The patient has a fever.)

⊿ **Simple Sentence 2:**

- "El paciente tiene tos".
  (The patient has a cough.)

⊿ **Compound Sentence:**

- "El paciente tiene fiebre **y** tos".
  *(The patient has a fever **and** a cough.)*

Combine the following sentences using 'pero':

- "El médico recomendó descanso".
  (The doctor recommended rest.)

- "El paciente tiene que trabajar".
  (The patient has to work.)

- "El médico recomendó descanso, pero el paciente tiene que trabajar".

Combine the following sentences using 'o':

- "Podemos administrar la vacuna hoy".
  (We can administer the vaccine today.)

- "Podemos programarla para la próxima semana".
  (We can schedule it for next week.)

- "Podemos administrar la vacuna hoy o podemos programarla para la próxima semana".

2. Constructing Complex Sentence

To add depth and clarity to explanations and instructions we can use more complex sentences. They often involve connectors like **'porque'** (because), **'cuando'** (when), and **'aunque'** (although), which provide additional details or reasoning.

Example:

Simple Sentence:

- "El paciente necesita medicamento".
  (The patient needs medication.)

Complex Sentence with 'porque':

- "El paciente necesita medicamento **porque** tiene una infección".
  *(The patient needs medication **because** they have an infection.)*

Combine the following sentences using 'cuando':

◢ **Simple Sentence 1:**

- "El paciente se siente mejor".
  (The patient feels better.)

◢ **Simple Sentence 2:**

- "El paciente toma su medicamento".
  (The patient takes their medication.)

- "El paciente se siente mejor **cuando** toma su medicamento".

Combine the following sentences using 'aunque':

◢ **Simple Sentence 1:**

- "El paciente tiene alergias severas".
  (The patient has severe allergies.)

◢ **Simple Sentence 2:**

- "El paciente puede recibir este tratamiento".
  (The patient can receive this treatment.)

- "El paciente tiene alergias severas **aunque** puede recibir este tratamiento".

FOUNDATIONAL SPANISH FOR HEALTHCARE

Think of this as your first step into a larger world, where you can greet, chat, and connect with your Spanish-speaking patients.

We're going to cover all the essentials you need - from 'Hola' to '¿Cómo te sientes?' - in a fun and friendly way.

Your Jumpstart to Speaking Spanish with Patients!

Mastering 'This', 'That', 'These', and 'Those'

1. **"This" in Spanish:**

    ◢ Este (eh-steh) for masculine nouns.
    ◢ Esta (eh-stah) for feminine nouns.

Examples:

    ◢ Este termómetro es nuevo. (This thermometer is new.)
    ◢ Esta receta es para el paciente. (This prescription is for the patient.)

2. **"That" in Spanish:**

    ◢ Ese (eh-seh) for masculine nouns.
    ◢ Esa (eh-sah) for feminine nouns.

Examples:

    ◢ Ese paciente necesita ayuda. (That patient needs help.)
    ◢ Esa silla de ruedas es para la sala de emergencias. (That wheelchair is for the emergency room.)

3. **"These" in Spanish:**

⊿ Estos (eh-stohs) for masculine nouns.
⊿ Estas (eh-stahs) for feminine nouns.

Examples:

⊿ Estos guantes son para la cirugía. (These gloves are for the surgery.)
⊿ Estas pastillas son para el dolor. (These pills are for the pain.)

4. **"Those" in Spanish:**

⊿ Esos (eh-sohs) for masculine nouns.
⊿ Esas (eh-sahs) for feminine nouns.

Examples:

⊿ Esos informes son del laboratorio. (Those reports are from the laboratory.)
⊿ Esas muletas están en la habitación 5. (Those crutches are in room 5.)

By practicing these words in everyday situations, you can quickly improve your ability to describe and refer to objects and people in Spanish. Remember, the key is to match the gender of the noun with the correct form of "this," "that," "these," or "those."

Basic Greetings & Farewells

1. **Buenos días** (Bwe-nos dee-ahs)

    ▪ Good morning

2. **Buenas tardes** (Bwe-nas tar-des)

    ▪ Good afternoon

3. **Buenas noches** (Bwe-nas noh-ches)

    ▪ Good night

4. **Hola** (Oh-lah)

   - Hello

5. **Adiós** (Ah-dee-ohs)

   - Goodbye

6. **Hasta luego** (Ah-sta loo-eh-go)

   - See you later

7. **Hasta mañana** (Ah-sta mah-nyah-nah)

   - See you tomorrow

8. **¿Cómo está?** (Coh-moh es-tah)

   - How are you? (formal)

9. **¿Cómo estás?** (Coh-moh es-tahs)

   - How are you? (informal)

10. **Mucho gusto** (Moo-choh goos-toh)

    - Nice to meet you

11. **Encantado/a** (En-cahn-tah-doh/dah)

    - Pleased to meet you

12. ¿Qué tal? (Keh tal)

- What's up?

_____

13. ¿Cómo va todo? (Coh-moh vah toh-doh)

- How is everything going?

_____

Practical Application

1. If you meet a Spanish-speaking patient for the first time in the afternoon, which greeting should you use?

_____

2. What phrase would you use to say goodbye to a patient you plan to see again tomorrow?

_____

3. How would you ask a new patient about their well-being in a formal manner?

_____

Answers

1. **If you meet a Spanish-speaking patient for the first time in the afternoon, which greeting should you use?**

    Answer: Use "Buenas tardes" (Good afternoon).

2. **What phrase would you use to say goodbye to a patient you plan to see again tomorrow?**

    Answer: Use "Hasta mañana" (See you tomorrow).

3. **How would you ask a new patient about their well-being in a formal manner?**

    Answer: Ask "¿Cómo está usted?" (How are you? - formal).
    The use of "usted" makes the question formal.

Symptoms & Conditions

1. **Fiebre** (Fee-eh-breh)

   - Fever

2. **Dolor** (Doh-lohr)

   - Pain

3. **Alergia** (Ahl-air-hee-ah)

   - Allergy

4. **Tos** (Tohs)

   - Cough

5. **Náuseas** (Nau-seh-ahs)

   - Nausea

6. **Diarrea** (Dee-ah-rreh-ah)

   - Diarrhea

7. **Estreñimiento** (Ehs-tren-yee-mee-en-toh)

   - Constipation

8. **Mareo** (Mah-reh-oh)

   - Dizziness

9. **Fatiga** (Fah-tee-gah)

   - Fatigue

   _____

10. **Sangrado** (Sahn-grah-doh)

    - Bleeding

    _____

Practical Application

1. What Spanish term would you use for a patient experiencing an elevated body temperature?

   _____

2. If a patient complains of discomfort in their stomach, which Spanish word is most appropriate to describe this symptom?

   _____

3. How would you refer to an adverse reaction to certain foods or environments in Spanish?

   _____

Answers

1. **What Spanish term would you use for a patient experiencing an elevated body temperature?**

    Answer: "Fiebre" (Fever).

2. **If a patient complains of discomfort in their stomach, which Spanish word is most appropriate to describe this symptom?**

    Answer: "Dolor" (Pain).

3. **How would you refer to an adverse reaction to certain foods or environments in Spanish?**

    Answer: "Alergia" (Allergy).

Body Parts

1. **Cabeza** (Kah-beh-sah)

   - Head

2. **Corazón** (Koh-rah-sohn)

   - Heart

3. **Estómago** (Ehs-toh-mah-goh)

   - Stomach

4. **Brazo** (Brah-soh)

   - Arm

5. **Pierna** (Pyehr-nah)

   - Leg

6. **Mano** (Mah-noh)

   - Hand

7. **Pie** (Pee-eh)

   - Foot

8. **Espalda** (Ehs-pahl-dah)

   - Back

9. **Pecho** (Peh-choh)

- Chest

_____

10. **Ojo** (Oh-hoh)

- Eye

_____

11. **Rodilla** (Roh-dee-yah)

- Knee

_____

12. **Cuello** (Kweh-yoh)

- Neck

_____

13. **Hombro** (Ohm-broh)

- Shoulder

_____

14. **Codo** (Koh-doh)

- Elbow

_____

15. **Muñeca** (Moo-nyeh-kah)

- Wrist

_____

16. **Tobillo** (Toh-bee-yoh)

- Ankle

_____

17. Dedo (Deh-doh)

- Finger

_____

18. Dedo del pie (Deh-doh del pee-eh)

- Toe

_____

19. Cadera (Kah-deh-rah)

- Hip

_____

20. Oreja (Oh-ray-hah)

- Ear

_____

Practical Application

1. What is the Spanish term for the body part that pumps blood?

_____

2. If a patient is experiencing discomfort in their lower limb, what Spanish word would you use to refer to that part of the body?

_____

3. How would you say "wrist" in Spanish, a common area for sprains?

_____

Answers

1. **What is the Spanish term for the body part that pumps blood?**
   Answer: "Corazón" (Heart).

2. **If a patient is experiencing discomfort in their lower limb, what Spanish word would you use to refer to that part of the body?**
   Answer: "Pierna" (Leg).

3. **How would you say "wrist" in Spanish, a common area for sprains?**
   Answer: "Muñeca" (Wrist).

Medical Procedures

1. **Examen** (Eks-ah-men)

   - Exam

2. **Cirugía** (Seer-roo-hee-ah)

   - Surgery

3. **Inyección** (Een-yek-see-on)

   - Injection

4. **Radiografía** (Rah-dee-oh-grah-fee-ah)

   - X-ray

5. **Ultrasonido** (Ool-trah-soh-nee-doh)

   - Ultrasound

6. **Análisis de sangre** (Ah-nah-lee-sees deh sahn-greh)

   - Blood test

7. **Vacunación** (Bah-koo-nah-see-ohn)

   - Vaccination

8. **Transfusión de sangre** (Trans-foo-see-on deh sahn-greh)

   - Blood transfusion

9. **Biopsia** (Bee-op-see-ah)

   - Biopsy

   _____

10. **Diálisis** (Dee-ah-lee-sees)

    - Dialysis

    _____

Practical Application

1. If a doctor takes a sample of tissue for examination, what is the Spanish term for this procedure?

    _____

2. The Spanish term for using high-frequency sound waves to image the body's interior, often in pregnancy.

    _____

3. A procedure where blood is transferred from one person to another, what is this called in Spanish?

    _____

1. **If a doctor takes a sample of tissue for examination, what is the Spanish term for this procedure?**

    Answer: The Spanish term for this procedure is "Biopsia" (Biopsy).

2. **The Spanish term for using high-frequency sound waves to image the body's interior, often in pregnancy.**

    Answer: "Ultrasonido" (Ultrasound)

3. **A procedure where blood is transferred from one person to another, what is this called in Spanish?**

    Answer: "Transfusión de sangre" (Blood transfusion)

Instructions & Responses

1. **Respire hondo** (Res-pee-reh hohn-doh)
   - Take a deep breath

2. **Relájese** (Reh-lah-heh-seh)
   - Relax (formal)

3. **Relájate** (Reh-lah-hah-teh)
   - Relax (informal)

4. **¿Entiende?** (En-tyen-deh?)
   - Do you understand? (formal)

5. **¿Entiendes?** (En-tyen-des?)
   - Do you understand? (informal)

6. **Por favor, siéntese** (Por fah-vor, see-ehn-teh-seh)
   - Please, sit down (formal)

7. **Por favor, siéntate** (Por fah-vor, see-ehn-tah-teh)
   - Please, sit down (informal)

8. **Necesito tomar su presión** (Neh-seh-see-toh toh-mar soo preh-see-on)
   - I need to take your blood pressure

9. **Vamos a hacer una prueba** (vah-mos ah ah-ser oo-nah prweh-bah)

   - We are going to do a test

   _____

10. **Mantenga la calma** (Mahn-ten-gah lah kahl-mah)

   - Keep calm

   _____

Practical Application

1. How would you ask a patient formally if they understand your instructions?

   _____

2. If a patient appears anxious and you want to tell them informally to calm down, what Spanish phrase would you use?

   _____

3. What would you say in Spanish if you need to inform a patient that you're going to conduct a test?

   _____

Answers

1. **How would you ask a patient formally if they understand your instructions?**

   Answer: "¿Entiende?" (Do you understand?)

2. **If a patient appears anxious and you want to tell them informally to calm down, what Spanish phrase would you use?**

   Answer: "Relájate" (Relax)

3. **What would you say in Spanish if you need to inform a patient that you're going to conduct a test?**

   Answer: "Vamos a hacer una prueba" (We are going to do a test)

Emergency Terms

1. **Emergencia** (Eh-mehr-hen-see-ah)

   - Emergency

     _____

2. **Urgente** (Oor-hen-teh)

   - Urgent

     _____

3. **Socorro** (Soh-kohr-roh)

   - Help

     _____

4. **Auxilio** (Ow-ksee-lee-oh)

   - Assistance

     _____

5. **Peligro** (Peh-lee-groh)

   - Danger

     _____

6. **Evacuar** (Eh-vah-koo-ahr)

   - Evacuate

     _____

7. **Primeros auxilios** (Pree-meh-ros owk-see-lee-ohs)

   - First aid

     _____

8. **Riesgo** (Ree-ess-goh)

   - Risk

     _____

9. **Contagio** (Kohn-tah-hee-oh)

   - Contagion

   _____

10. **Desmayo** (Des-mah-yoh)

    - Fainting

    _____

Practical Application

1. What Spanish term would you use to indicate an immediate, critical situation in the hospital?

   _____

2. If someone is in danger and needs immediate assistance, what word should you shout?

   _____

3. How would you refer to 'first aid' in Spanish during a medical emergency?

   _____

Answers

1. **What Spanish term would you use to indicate an immediate, critical situation in the hospital?**

   Answer: "Emergencia" (Emergency)

2. **If someone is in danger and needs immediate assistance, what word should you shout?**

   Answer: "Socorro" (Help)

3. **How would you refer to 'first aid' in Spanish during a medical emergency?**

   Answer: "Primeros auxilios" (First aid)

Pharmacy Terms

1. **Medicamento** (Meh-dee-kah-men-toh)

   ▪ Medication

2. **Receta** (Reh-seh-tah)

   ▪ Prescription

3. **Dosis** (Doh-sees)

   ▪ Dose

4. **Farmacéutico/a** (Fahr-mah-seh-oo-tee-koh/ah)

   ▪ Pharmacist

5. **Antibiótico** (An-tee-bee-oh-tee-koh)

   ▪ Antibiotic

6. **Efectos secundarios** (Eh-fehk-tos seh-koon-dah-ree-ohs)

   ▪ Side effects

7. **Pastillas** (Pahs-tee-yahs)

   ▪ Pills

8. **Jarabe** (Hah-rah-beh)

   ▪ Syrup

9. **Instrucciones de uso** (Een-struk-see-oh-nes deh oo-soh)

   ▪ Directions for use

   _____

10. **Fecha de caducidad** (Feh-chah deh kah-doo-see-dahd)

   ▪ Expiration date

   _____

Practical Application

1. How do you say 'antibiotic' in Spanish, a common type of medication?

   _____

2. What is the Spanish term for 'side effects' that patients should be aware of?

   _____

3. If you are giving a patient 'directions for use' of a medication, what phrase would you use in Spanish?

   _____

Answers

1. **How do you say 'antibiotic' in Spanish, a common type of medication?**

    Answer: "Antibiótico" (Antibiotic)

2. **What is the Spanish term for 'side effects' that patients should be aware of?**

    Answer: "Efectos secundarios" (Side effects)

3. **If you are giving a patient 'directions for use' of a medication, what phrase would you use in Spanish?**

    Answer: "Instrucciones de uso" (Directions for use)

General Healthcare Terms

1. **Sangre** (Sahn-greh)
   - Blood

2. **Presión arterial** (Preh-see-ohn ar-teh-ree-ahl)
   - Blood pressure

3. **Diagnóstico** (Dee-ahg-nos-tee-koh)
   - Diagnosis

4. **Vacuna** (Bah-koo-nah)
   - Vaccine

5. **Salud** (Sah-lood)
   - Health

6. **Paciente** (Pah-see-en-teh)
   - Patient

7. **Síntomas** (Seen-toh-mahs)
   - Symptoms

8. **Enfermedad** (En-fer-meh-dahd)
   - Illness

9. **Recuperación** (Reh-koo-peh-rah-see-ohn)

   - Recovery

   _____

10. **Examen físico** (Eks-ah-men fees-ee-koh)

   - Physical exam

   _____

Practical Application

1. What Spanish term refers to the overall wellness or well-being of a person?

   _____

2. How would you say 'vaccine' in Spanish, especially important in immunization contexts?

   _____

3. If a doctor is conducting a 'physical exam' on a patient, what is this called in Spanish?

   _____

Answers

1. **What Spanish term refers to the overall wellness or well-being of a person?**

   Answer: "Salud" (Health)

2. **How would you say 'vaccine' in Spanish, especially important in immunization contexts?**

   Answer: "Vacuna" (Vaccine)

3. **If a doctor is conducting a 'physical exam' on a patient, what is this called in Spanish?**

   Answer: "Examen físico" (Physical exam)

Patient Care

1. **Reposo en cama** (Reh-poh-soh en kah-mah)

   - Bed rest

   _____

2. **Historial clínico** (Ees-toh-ree-ahl kleen-ee-koh)

   - Medical history

   _____

3. **Tratamiento** (Trah-tah-mee-en-toh)

   - Treatment

   _____

4. **Cuidado** (Kwee-dah-doh)

   - Care

   _____

5. **Alta médica** (Ahl-tah meh-dee-kah)

   - Medical discharge

   _____

6. **Consentimiento informado** (Kohn-sen-tee-mee-en-toh een-for-mah-doh)

   - Informed consent

   _____

7. **Cuidados paliativos** (Kwee-dah-dohs pah-lee-ah-tee-vohs)

   - Palliative care

   _____

8. **Plan de cuidados** (Plahn deh kwee-dah-dohs)

   - Care plan

   _____

9. **Terapia** (Teh-rah-pee-ah)

   - Therapy

     _____

10. **Seguimiento** (Seh-ghee-mee-en-toh)

    - Follow-up

      _____

Practical Application

1. What is the term for 'palliative care' in Spanish, which focuses on comfort for serious illness?

   _____

2. If a patient is given 'informed consent' to sign, what is this called in Spanish?

   _____

3. How do you say 'follow-up' in Spanish, referring to subsequent medical appointments or checks?

   _____

Answers

1. **What is the term for 'palliative care' in Spanish, which focuses on comfort for serious illness?**

   Answer: "Cuidados paliativos" (Palliative care)

2. **If a patient is given 'informed consent' to sign, what is this called in Spanish?**

   Answer: "Consentimiento informado" (Informed consent)

3. **How do you say 'follow-up' in Spanish, referring to subsequent medical appointments or checks?**

   Answer: "Seguimiento" (Follow-up)

Common Illnesses

1. **Gripe** (Gree-peh)

   - Flu

2. **Diarrea** (Dee-ah-rreh-ah)

   - Diarrhea

3. **Asma** (Ahs-mah)

   - Asthma

4. **Varicela** (Vah-ree-seh-lah)

   - Chickenpox

5. **Hipertensión** (Ee-per-ten-see-ohn)

   - Hypertension

6. **Bronquitis** (Bron-kee-tees)

   - Bronchitis

7. **Insomnio** (Een-sohm-nee-oh)

   - Insomnia

8. **Apendicitis** (Ah-pen-dee-see-tees)

   - Appendicitis

9. **Anemia** (Ah-neh-mee-ah)

- Anemia

_____

Practical Application

1. What Spanish term is used for a respiratory condition characterized by wheezing and shortness of breath?

_____

2. How do you say 'chickenpox' in Spanish, a common viral illness in children?

_____

3. If a patient has elevated blood pressure, what is this condition called in Spanish?

_____

Answers

1. **What Spanish term is used for a respiratory condition characterized by wheezing and shortness of breath?**

    Answer: "Asma" (Asthma)

2. **How do you say 'chickenpox' in Spanish, a common viral illness in children?**

    Answer: "Varicela" (Chickenpox)

3. **If a patient has elevated blood pressure, what is this condition called in Spanish?**

    Answer: "Hipertensión" (Hypertension)

Common Greetings - Formal and Informal

◢ **Formal:**

- **Buenos días, señor / señora [last name]**
  (Good morning, Mr. / Mrs. [last name])

- **"Buenas tardes, doctora / doctor [last name]"**
  (Good afternoon, Doctor [last name])

- **"Buenos días, ¿cómo amaneció?"**
  (Good morning, how did you wake up?)

◢ **Informal:**

- **"Hola, ¿cómo te va?"**
  (Hi, how's it going?)

- **"¿Qué tal?"**
  (What's up?)

- **"¡Hola! ¿Qué pasa?"**
  (Hey! What's happening?).

Using Polite Forms:

- **"¿Cómo está usted?"**
  (How are you? - formal)

  _____

Vs.

- **"¿Cómo estás?"**
  (How are you? - informal)

  _____

Patient-Specific Greetings:

For children:

- **"Hola, campeón/campeona"**
  (Hello, little champ)

  _____

- **"¡Hola a todos, ¿cómo están el día de hoy?"**
  (Hello everyone, how are you today?)

  _____

For elderly patients:

- **"Buenos días, don/doña [name]"**
  (Good morning, Mr./Mrs. [name])

  _____

Farewells and Wishing Well:

General farewell:

- **"Hasta la próxima"**
  (Until next time)

  _____

- **"Que tenga un buen día"**
  (Have a good day)

◢ **Wishing well:**

- **"Espero que se sienta mejor"**
  (I hope you feel better)

- **"Siga las indicaciones y mejórese pronto".**
  (Follow the instructions and get well soon).

Cultural Nuances

1. **Respectful Addressing:**
   - When speaking to elderly or first-time patients, use formal titles.

     Example: Greet with 'Buenos días, señor Rodríguez' instead of just 'Buenos días.' This shows respect and professionalism.

2. **Use of 'Hasta luego':**
   - In many Latin American countries, 'Hasta luego' is preferred over 'Adiós' for farewells, as it's friendlier.

     Example: End an appointment with 'Hasta luego, nos vemos en su próxima cita' to convey warmth.

3. **Titles and Formality:**
   - Address fellow healthcare professionals by their titles.

     For example: introduce a nurse as 'Le presento a la enfermera López'.

4. **Variations in Vocabulary:**

   Be aware of regional differences in words to ensure accurate communication.

   - For instance, **'coger'** is common in Spain for 'to take,' but in Latin America, use **'tomar'** to avoid misunderstandings."

- **Emergency Room:** In some Latin American countries, it's referred to as "Sala de urgencias," while in Spain, it's known as "Urgencias" or "Emergencias."
- **Bandage:** In many Latin American countries, a bandage is called "venda," whereas in Spain, it's often referred to as "tirita."
- **Shot/Injection:** The common term in Latin America is "inyección," but in Spain, it's also known as "pinchazo."

5. **Informal Language:**

- With younger, familiar patients, it's okay to be more informal.

  > **Example:** Greet a regular teenage patient with '¿Qué tal, Carlos? ¿Cómo has estado?'
  > *How are you, Carlos? How have you been?*

Practical Application

1. How do you say "Good morning" in Spanish when addressing an elderly patient formally?

   _____

2. Translate "See you later" into Spanish, as commonly used in Latin America.

   _____

3. Choose the informal way to ask "How are you?" in Spanish.

   _____

4. What is the Spanish phrase for "Take care" used as a farewell to a patient?

   _____

5. If you were greeting a group of children in a Spanish-speaking setting, which phrase would you use?

   _____

1. **How do you say "Good morning" in Spanish when addressing an elderly patient formally?**

    Answer: "Buenos días, don/doña [name]" (Good morning, Mr./Mrs. [name])

2. **Translate "See you later" into Spanish, as commonly used in Latin America.**

    Answer: "Hasta luego" (See you later)

3. **Choose the informal way to ask "How are you?" in Spanish.**

    Answer: "¿Cómo estás?" (How are you?)

4. **What is the Spanish phrase for "Take care" used as a farewell to a patient?**

    Answer: "Cuídese" (Take care)

5. **If you were greeting a group of children in a Spanish-speaking setting, which phrase could you use?**

    Answer: "¡Hola a todos, ¿cómo están el día de hoy?"
    (Hello everyone, how are you today?)

Healthcare Communication Essentials:
EXPLAINING ROLES, ASKING PATIENT DETAILS, PRIVACY AND CONSENT

In this section, we'll go through the essentials of introducing yourself and your role in healthcare, collecting vital patient information, and discussing confidentiality and consent. This knowledge is crucial for fostering trust with Spanish-speaking patients. You'll practice inquiring about names, dates of birth, and medical history in Spanish, and gain the skills to reassure patients regarding the security of their information. We'll also delve into the art of obtaining consent for treatments or procedures. It's all about effective and respectful communication in medical settings.

Explaining Professional Roles

Clear communication of your job and responsibilities sets the stage for effective patient care. Below are some phrases to help you convey this information professionally, yet in a way that's easy for patients to understand. It's a key step in building a comfortable and reassuring environment for them.

1. **Practical Examples:**

    A. **"Soy enfermero/enfermera, voy a tomar su presión arterial".**
    (I am a nurse, I am going to take your blood pressure.)

    B. **"Como su médico, revisaré sus resultados de laboratorio".**
    (As your doctor, I will review your lab results.)

C. **"Soy fisioterapeuta y le ayudaré con su rehabilitación".**
   (I am the physiotherapist and will help with your rehabilitation.)

   _____

D. **"Como farmacéutico, le explicaré cómo tomar estos medicamentos".**
   (As a pharmacist, I will explain how to take these medications.)

   _____

2. Pronunciation Practice:

⊿ Focus on pronouncing roles correctly:

   i.   Enfermero/enfermera (ehn-fer-meh-ro/ehn-fer-meh-rah)
   ii. Médico/médica (meh-dee-koh/meh-dee-kah)
   iii. Fisioterapeuta (fee-see-oh-teh-rah-peh-oo-tah)
   iv. Farmacéutico (fahr-mah-seh-oo-tee-koh)

⊿ Repeat the sentences, emphasizing the job title.

3. Role-Play Scenarios:

Scenario A: Introducing Yourself - Start with your name and role, followed by a brief explanation of how you'll assist the patient.

> **Example:** "Hola, me llamo [Your Name] y soy el/la [Your Role].
> Estoy aquí para [brief description of your assistance]."

> **Translation:** "Hello, my name is [Your Name], and I am the [Your Role].
> I am here to [brief description of your assistance]."

Scenario B: Explain your role in a patient's treatment plan.

> **Example:** "Como [Your Role], mi responsabilidad es [describe a key aspect of your role in the treatment plan]."

> **Translation:** "As a [Your Role], my responsibility is to [describe a key aspect of your role in the treatment plan]."

Asking for Patient Details

Having a set of clear questions for gathering their details is very helpful. These questions are perfect for getting essential info like names, birth dates, and health backgrounds. They're designed to make your interactions smooth and ensure your patients feel heard and understood while making sure you have the information needed to provide excellent care.

1. **Practical Examples:**

    A. **"¿Cómo se llama?"**
        (What is your name?)

    B. **"¿Cuál es su fecha de nacimiento?"**
        (What is your date of birth?)

    C. **"¿Tiene alguna alergia?"**
        (Do you have any allergies?)

    D. **"¿Cuál es su historial médico?"**
        (What is your medical history?)

    E. **"¿Qué medicamentos está tomando actualmente?"**
        (What medications are you currently taking?)

    F. **"¿Cuál es su dirección actual?"**
        (What is your current address?)

    G. **"¿Cuál es su número de teléfono?"**
        (What is your phone number?)

    H. **"¿Hay alguna condición médica que debamos conocer?"**
        (Is there any medical condition we should know about?)

I. **"¿Cómo podemos comunicarnos con su contacto de emergencia?"**
(How can we contact your emergency person?)

2. **Pronunciation Practice:**

   ◢ Focus on clear pronunciation of key questions.

   ◢ Repeat each question, paying attention to the intonation and rhythm.

   ◢ Practice saying each question slowly, then at a normal speaking pace.

   ◢ Focus on the pronunciation of key words like:

   - "Dirección" (dee-rehk-see-ohn)
   - "Teléfono" (teh-leh-foh-noh)

3. **Role-Play Scenarios:**

   Scenario A:

   You're a nurse collecting patient information at check-in.

   Ask for their name, date of birth, and if they have any current health concerns.

   Begin with: "Buenos días, necesito hacerle algunas preguntas para su registro".

   Scenario B:

   As a doctor, you're taking a patient's medical history.

   Inquire about their medical history, current medications, and if they have any allergies.

   Start with: "Voy a revisar su historial médico. Comencemos con su nombre y edad".

Discussing Privacy

You will find these phrases to be really useful when you need to talk about keeping things private with your Spanish-speaking patients. They give you a lot of different ways to express the importance of confidentiality and making sure your patients feel their information is safe with you.

1. **Practical Examples:**

    A. **"Protegemos su información".**
    (We protect your information.)

    B. **"Su privacidad es importante".**
    (Your privacy is important.)

    C. **"¿Me permite compartir esta información?"**
    (Can you give me permission to share this information?)

    D. **"Sus datos son confidenciales".**
    (Your data is confidential.)

    E. **"Sólo usaremos su información para su cuidado".**
    (We will only use your information for your care.)

    F. **"¿Está de acuerdo en compartir su historial médico con nosotros?"**
    (Are you comfortable sharing your medical history with us?)

    G. **"Protegemos su información personal".**
    (Your personal information is handled with care.)

    H. **"Nuestro personal está entrenado en privacidad y confidencialidad".**
    (Our staff is trained in privacy and confidentiality.)

I. **"Le informaremos antes de usar su información para cualquier propósito".**
(We will inform you before using your information for any purpose.)

J. **"¿Tiene preguntas sobre cómo protegemos su información?"**
(Do you have questions about how we protect your information?)

2. **Pronunciation Practice:**

⊿ Emphasize key phrases like "confidencialidad" (kohn-fee-den-see-ahl-ee-dahd) and "consentimiento" (kohn-sen-tee-mee-en-toh).

⊿ Practice these sentences, focusing on clarity and a tone of assurance.

3. **Role-Play Scenarios:**

Scenario A: Assuring a New Patient About Data Confidentiality

Start with:

"Buenos días. Su información está a salvo".
(Good morning. Your information is safe.)

Continue:

"Todos aquí protegen su privacidad".
(Everyone here protects your privacy.)

Scenario B: Discussing Consent for Information Sharing

Start with:

"Para compartir su información, necesitamos su permiso".
(To share your information, we need your permission.)

Continue:

"¿Está de acuerdo?"
(Do you agree?)

Obtaining Consent

Let's cover key phrases to ensure patients understand and agree to procedures or treatments.

1. **Practical Examples:**

   A. **"Es importante que entienda los detalles del procedimiento".**
   (It's important that you understand the details of the procedure.)

   _____

   B. **"¿Puede firmar aquí para indicar que está de acuerdo?"**
   (Can you sign here to show your agreement?)

   _____

   C. **"¿Ha entendido todos los riesgos y beneficios del tratamiento?"**
   (Have you understood all the risks and benefits of the treatment?)

   _____

   D. **"Su firma aquí confirma que ha recibido toda la información necesaria".**
   (Your signature here confirms that you have received all the necessary information.)

   _____

   E. **"¿Entiende los efectos secundarios posibles?"**
   (Do you understand the possible side effects?)

   _____

   F. **"Por favor, lea este documento antes de dar su aprobación".**
   (Please read this document before giving your approval.)

   _____

   G. **"Es su derecho hacer preguntas antes de dar su consentimiento".**
   (It is your right to ask questions before consenting.)

   _____

   H. **"¿Está de acuerdo con la información proporcionada?"**
   (Are you comfortable with the information provided?)

   _____

I. **"Firme aquí si está de acuerdo con los procedimientos descritos".**
(Sign here if you agree with the described procedures.)

J. **"Su consentimiento informado es esencial para nosotros".**
(Your informed consent is essential to us.)

K. **"¿Comprende lo que implica este tratamiento?"**
(Do you understand what this treatment involves?)

L. **"Vamos a explicarle cada paso del procedimiento".**
(We will explain each step of the procedure to you.)

M. **"¿Tiene alguna inquietud que quiera discutir?"**
(Do you have any concerns you would like to discuss?)

N. **"Estamos aquí para responder todas sus preguntas".**
(We are here to answer all your questions.)

2. **Pronunciation Practice:**

⊿ **Focus on key terms like:**

"Consentimiento" (kohn-sen-tee-mee-en-toh)

"Procedimiento" (proh-seh-dee-mee-en-toh)

⊿ Repeat each sentence, emphasizing clarity and intonation to convey the importance of understanding and agreement.

3. **Role-Play Scenarios:**

Scenario A: Explaining a consent form for a surgery.

Start with:

"Antes de la cirugía, firme el consentimiento aquí".
(Before the surgery, sign the consent here.)

Continue:

"¿Entiende los detalles?"
(Do you understand the details?)

Scenario B: Discussing a new treatment plan.

Start with:

"Vamos a hablar sobre su nuevo plan de tratamiento".
(Let's talk about your new treatment plan.)

Continue:

"¿Está de acuerdo con estos pasos?"
(Do you agree with these steps?)

Conclusion

And that's a wrap on the basics of Spanish for healthcare! With these foundational skills in your toolkit, you're well on your way to creating strong, meaningful connections with your Spanish-speaking patients.

Every 'Buenos días' and '¿Cómo está?' you share is more than just words; it's a bridge to better care and stronger patient relationships. Keep practicing what you've learned, stay curious about the language, and don't be afraid to experiment with your new skills in real conversations.

The journey to fluency is a marathon, not a sprint, and you're off to a fantastic start. Soon, you'll be chatting away with confidence and making a real difference in your patients' lives.

Medical Vocabulary and Key Phrases

In this section we'll learn everyday medical words and phrases, with topics like handling pain, gastrointestinal issues, chronic conditions, cardiology, mental well-being, comfort, and instructions. You'll practice by translating real-life situations, chatting in simple dialogues, and picking up interesting cultural tidbits. Don't worry; we'll have quick recaps to help you remember it all!

Pain

DESCRIPTORS

1. **Agudo** (ah-goo-doh):

   Sharp

2. **Sordo** (sohr-doh):

   Dull

3. **Punzante** (poon-sahn-teh):

   Stabbing

4. **Ardor** (ahr-dohr):

   Burning

5. **Latente** (lah-ten-teh):

   Throbbing

6. **Cólico** (koh-lee-koh):

Colicky

7. **Irradiado** (ee-rah-dee-ah-doh):

Radiating

8. **Hormigueo** (or-mee-geh-oh):

Tingling

9. **Opresivo** (oh-preh-see-voh):

Pressing

10. **Calambres** (kah-lahm-bres):

Cramps

11. **Lacerante** (lah-seh-rahn-teh):

Lacerating

12. **Molestia** (moh-les-tee-ah):

Discomfort

1. **Constante** (kohn-stahn-teh):

   Constant

   _____

2. **Intermitente** (een-ter-mee-ten-teh):

   Intermittent

   _____

3. **Ocasional** (oh-kah-see-oh-nahl):

   Occasional

   _____

4. **Frecuente** (freh-kwen-teh):

   Frequent

   _____

5. **Permanente** (pehr-mah-nen-teh):

   Permanent

   _____

6. **Recurrente** (reh-koo-rren-teh):

   Recurring

   _____

7. **Esporádico** (es-poh-rah-dee-koh):

   Sporadic

   _____

8. **Continuo** (kohn-tee-noo-oh):

   Continuous

   _____

1. **Cabeza** (kah-beh-sah):

   Head
   _____

2. **Espalda** (ehs-pahl-dah):

   Back
   _____

3. **Abdomen** (ahb-doh-men):

   Abdomen
   _____

4. **Pecho** (peh-choh):

   Chest
   _____

5. **Rodilla** (roh-dee-yah):

   Knee
   _____

6. **Hombro** (ohm-broh):

   Shoulder
   _____

7. **Articulaciones** (ar-tee-koo-lah-see-oh-nes):

   Joints
   _____

8. **Tobillo** (toh-bee-yoh):

   Ankle
   _____

9. **Cuello** (kweh-yoh):

Neck

10. **Brazo** (brah-soh):

Arm

11. **Muslo** (moos-loh):

Thigh

12. **Cadera** (kah-deh-rah):

Hip

13. **Muñeca** (moo-nyeh-kah):

Wrist

14. **Torso** (tor-soh):

Torso

Practical Examples

A. **"¿El dolor es constante durante todo el día?"**
(Is the pain constant throughout the day?)

_____

B. **"¿El dolor aumenta con el movimiento?"**
(Does the pain increase with movement?)

_____

C. **"¿Siente el dolor sólo en un lado del cuerpo?"**
(Do you feel the pain on only one side of the body?)

_____

D. **"¿Cómo describiría el dolor en una escala del 1 al 10?"**
(How would you describe the pain on a scale of 1 to 10?)

_____

E. **"¿El dolor se irradia a otras partes del cuerpo?"**
(Does the pain radiate to other parts of the body?)

_____

F. **"¿Ha tomado algo para aliviar el dolor?"**
(Have you taken anything to alleviate the pain?)

_____

G. **"¿Tiene otros síntomas además del dolor?"**
(Do you have any other symptoms besides the pain?)

_____

H. **"¿El dolor comenzó de repente o gradualmente?"**
(Did the pain start suddenly or gradually?)

_____

I. **"¿Hay algo que mejore o empeore el dolor?"**
(Is there anything that improves or worsens the pain?)

_____

J. "¿El dolor le impide realizar sus actividades diarias?"
(Does the pain prevent you from doing your daily activities?)

_____

K. "¿Ha tenido este tipo de dolor antes?"
(Have you had this type of pain before?)

_____

L. "¿El dolor se siente como presión o ardor?"
(Does the pain feel like pressure or a burning sensation?)

_____

Translate That Scenario!

You'll be given a simple sentence or scenario in English related to pain. Your task is to do your best to translate it into Spanish, using the words and phrases you've learned.

Scenario 1: A patient complains of intermittent stabbing pain in their lower back.

_____

Scenario 2: A woman describes a throbbing headache that worsens at night.

_____

Scenario 3: A man mentions a dull ache in his knee after running.

_____

Scenario 4: A child says they have a sharp pain in their stomach after eating.

_____

Scenario 5: An elderly person reports feeling a constant burning sensation in their chest.

_____

Scenario 1: A patient complains of intermittent stabbing pain in their lower back.

Translation: "Un paciente se queja de dolor punzante intermitente en la espalda baja".

Scenario 2: A woman describes a throbbing headache that worsens at night.

Translation: "Una mujer describe un dolor de cabeza palpitante que empeora por la noche".

Scenario 3: A man mentions a dull ache in his knee after running.

Translation: "Un hombre menciona un dolor sordo en la rodilla después de correr".

Scenario 4: A child says they have a sharp pain in their stomach after eating.

Translation: "Un niño dice que tiene un dolor agudo en el estómago después de comer".

Scenario 5: An elderly person reports feeling a constant burning sensation in their chest.

Translation: "Una persona mayor informa que siente un ardor constante en el pecho".

Dialogue 1

- **Doctor:** "¿Dónde siente el dolor?"
- **Paciente:** "Siento un dolor punzante en mi hombro izquierdo".
- **Doctor:** «¿Es un dolor constante o intermitente?»
- **Paciente:** "Es intermitente, pero muy agudo cuando ocurre".

Comprehension Questions:

1. How does the patient describe the pain in their shoulder?

2. Which shoulder is affected by the pain?

3. Does the patient describe the pain as constant, or does it come and go?

English Translation:

- **Doctor:** "Where do you feel the pain?"
- **Patient:** "I feel a stabbing pain in my left shoulder."
- **Doctor:** "Is the pain constant or intermittent?"
- **Patient:** "It's intermittent, but very sharp when it happens."

Dialogue 2

- **Enfermera:** «¿Cómo describiría su dolor de cabeza?»
- **Paciente:** "Es un dolor sordo y constante".
- **Enfermera:** «¿Ha experimentado esto antes?»
- **Paciente:** "Sí, usualmente cuando estoy estresado".

Comprehension Questions:

1. What type of headache does the patient describe?

2. Is the headache occasional or continuous?

3. What does the patient associate the headache with?

English Translation:

- **Nurse:** "How would you describe your headache?"
- **Patient:** "It's a dull and constant pain."
- **Nurse:** "Have you experienced this before?"
- **Patient:** "Yes, usually when I'm stressed."

Cultural Notes - Did You Know?

1. **Expressing Pain:** For example, in Mexico, patients might use vivid descriptions like "duele como si me estuvieran quemando" (it hurts as if I'm being burned), emphasizing the intensity.

2. **Traditional Remedies:** In some Andean cultures, patients might first try herbal teas (like 'mate de coca') for pain relief before seeking medical attention.

3. **Language Nuances:** The term "dolor" might be interpreted differently across regions. In Spain, "dolor fuerte" might be understood as severe pain, whereas in some Latin American countries, it might be considered moderate pain.

4. **Family Involvement:** In many Hispanic families, discussing pain and medical conditions often involves multiple family members, who may also describe the patient's pain based on observations.

True or False:

1. (True/False) "Dolor agudo" means dull pain.
2. (True/False) "Náuseas" translates to nausea in English.
3. (True/False) "Dolor constante" refers to intermittent pain.

How Do You Say?

1. Throbbing pain

    _____

2. I feel bloated

    _____

3. I have a headache

    _____

4. Back pain

    _____

Scenario Response:

A patient complains of a burning sensation in their stomach. What Spanish term describes this sensation?

_____

COMPREHENSION RECAP ANSWERS	
True or False:	**How Do You Say?**
1. False	1. **Dolor latente** - Throbbing pain
2. True	2. **Me siento hinchado/a** - I feel bloated
3. False	3. **Tengo dolor de cabeza** - I have a headache
	4. **Dolor de espalda** - Back pain

Scenario Response:

A patient complains of a burning sensation in their stomach. What Spanish term describes this sensation?

Una sensación de ardor en el estómago

Gastrointestinal

1. **Náuseas** (nau-seh-ahs):

   Nausea

2. **Acidez** (ah-see-dehs):

   Heartburn

3. **Diarrea** (dee-ah-reh-ah):

   Diarrhea

4. **Estreñimiento** (ehs-tren-yee-mee-en-toh):

   Constipation

5. **Hinchazón** (een-chah-sohn):

   Bloating

6. **Gases** (gah-sehs):

   Gas

7. **Vómito** (voh-mee-toh):

   Vomiting

8. **Cólicos** (koh-lee-kohs):

Cramps

9. **Indigestión** (een-dee-hes-tee-ohn):

Indigestion

10. **Pérdida de apetito** (pehr-dee-dah deh ah-peh-tee-toh):

Loss of appetite

11. **Ardor estomacal** (ahr-dohr es-toh-mah-kahl):

Stomach burning

12. **Reflujo** (reh-floo-hoh):

Reflux

DIET-RELATED

1. **Fibra** (fee-brah):

Fiber

2. **Hidratación** (ee-drah-tah-see-ohn):

Hydration

3. **Deshidratado/a** (deh-see-drah-tah-doh/dah)

Dehydrated

4. **Dieta blanda** (dee-eh-tah blahn-dah):

Soft diet

5. **Grasas** (grah-sahs):

Fats

6. **Proteínas** (proh-teh-ee-nahs):

Proteins

7. **Carbohidratos** (kahr-boh-ee-drah-tohs):

Carbohydrates

8. **Deslactosado/a** (dehs-lahk-toh-sah-doh/dah):

Lactose-free

9. **Bajo en sal** (bah-hoh ehn sahl):

Low-salt

10. **Alimentos integrales** (ah-lee-men-tohs een-teh-grah-lehs):

Whole foods

11. Comidas pequeñas (koh-mee-dahs peh-keh-nyahs):

Small meals

12. Evitar alcohol (eh-vee-tahr ahl-koh-ohl):

Avoid alcohol

13. Comer despacio (koh-mehr dehs-pah-see-oh):

Eat slowly

PATIENT INSTRUCTIONS

1. **Beber agua** (beh-behr ah-gwah):

   Drink water

2. **Evitar picante** (eh-vee-tahr pee-kahn-teh):

   Avoid spicy food

3. **Comer pequeñas porciones** (koh-mehr peh-keh-nyahs pohr-see-oh-nehs):

   Eat small portions

4. **Seguir una dieta equilibrada** (seh-geer oo-nah dee-eh-tah eh-kee-lee-brah-dah):

   Follow a balanced diet

3

5. **Descansar el estómago** (dehs-kahn-sahr ehl es-toh-mah-goh):

   Rest the stomach

6. **Tomar el medicamento con alimentos**

   (toh-mahr ehl meh-dee-kah-men-toh kohn ah-lee-men-tohs):

   Take medication with food

7. **Evitar comidas grasosas** (eh-vee-tahr koh-mee-dahs grah-soh-sahs):

   Avoid greasy foods

8. **Mantenerse hidratado** (mahn-teh-nehr-seh ee-drah-tah-doh):

   Stay hydrated

9. **Limitar el consumo de café** (lee-mee-tahr ehl kohn-soo-moh deh kah-feh):

   Limit coffee intake

10. **Aumentar el consumo de verduras**

    (ow-men-tahr ehl kohn-soo-moh deh behr-doo-rahs):

    Increase vegetable intake

11. **No comer demasiado rápido** (noh koh-mehr deh-mah-see-ah-doh rah-pee-doh):

    Do not eat too fast

12. **Incluir más frutas** (een-kloo-eer mahs froo-tahs):

Include more fruits

Practical Examples

1. **"¿Ha experimentado náuseas o vómitos recientemente?"**

   (Have you experienced nausea or vomiting recently?)

2. **"Recomiendo aumentar la ingesta de fibra para mejorar su digestión".**

   (I recommend increasing your fiber intake to improve your digestion.)

3. **"Evite alimentos grasosos para reducir la acidez".**

   (Avoid greasy foods to reduce heartburn.)

4. **"Para su estreñimiento, beba más agua y coma frutas".**

   (For your constipation, drink more water and eat fruits.)

5. **"¿Siente hinchazón después de comer ciertos alimentos?"**

   (Do you feel bloating after eating certain foods?)

6. **"Es importante mantenerse hidratado, especialmente si tiene diarrea".**

   (It's important to stay hydrated, especially if you have diarrhea.)

7. **"Una dieta baja en sal puede ayudar con su presión arterial".**

   (A low-salt diet can help with your blood pressure.)

   _____

8. **"Incluya más proteínas magras en sus comidas".**

   (Include more lean proteins in your meals.)

   _____

9. **"Limitar el café puede aliviar su indigestión".**

   (Limiting coffee may relieve your indigestion.)

   _____

10. **"¿Ha notado cólicos o gases después de las comidas?"**

    (Have you noticed cramps or gas after meals?)

    _____

11. **"Comer despacio y en porciones pequeñas puede mejorar su digestión".**

    (Eating slowly and in small portions can improve your digestion.)

    _____

12. **"Evite comidas picantes si sufre de reflujo".**

    (Avoid spicy foods if you suffer from reflux.)

    _____

Translate That Scenario!

You'll be given a simple sentence or scenario in English related to gastrointestinal issues. Your task is to do your best to translate it into Spanish, using the words and phrases you've learned.

Scenario 1: A patient complains of heartburn after eating spicy food.

_____

Scenario 2: Someone is experiencing bloating and gas.

_____

Scenario 3: A patient needs advice on a diet for managing constipation.

_____

Scenario 4: A person is describing their chronic indigestion issues.

_____

Scenario 5: A nurse advises a patient to stay hydrated due to frequent diarrhea.

_____

Scenario 1: A patient complains of heartburn after eating spicy food.

Translation: "Un paciente se queja de acidez después de comer comida picante".

Scenario 2: Someone is experiencing bloating and gas.

Translation: "Alguien experimenta hinchazón y gases".

Scenario 3: A patient needs advice on a diet for managing constipation.

Translation: "Un paciente necesita consejos sobre una dieta para manejar el estreñimiento".

Scenario 4: A person is describing their chronic indigestion issues.

Translation: "Una persona describe sus problemas crónicos de indigestión".

Scenario 5: A nurse advises a patient to stay hydrated due to frequent diarrhea.

Translation: "Una enfermera aconseja a un paciente mantenerse hidratado debido a la diarrea frecuente"

Dialogue 1

- **Enfermera**: "¿Cómo ha sido su apetito últimamente?"
- **Paciente**: "He tenido pérdida de apetito y acidez".
- **Enfermera**: "Le recomiendo evitar comidas picantes y grasosas".
- **Paciente**: "Entendido, seguiré sus consejos".

Comprehension Questions:

1. What symptom is the patient experiencing along with loss of appetite?
2. What does the nurse recommend the patient avoid?
3. Does the patient agree to follow the nurse's advice?

English Translation:

- **Nurse**: "How has your appetite been lately?"
- **Patient**: "I've had a loss of appetite and heartburn."
- **Nurse**: "I recommend you avoid spicy and greasy foods."
- **Patient**: "Understood, I'll follow your advice."

Dialogue 2

- **Doctor**: "¿Ha experimentado diarrea o estreñimiento?"
- **Paciente**: "Sí, he tenido diarrea frecuente".
- **Doctor**: "Es importante mantenerse hidratado. Beba mucha agua".
- **Paciente**: "Gracias, lo haré".

Comprehension Questions:

1. What gastrointestinal issue is the patient currently experiencing?
2. What does the doctor advise the patient to do to manage this issue?
3. How does the patient respond to the doctor's advice?

English Translation:

- **Doctor**: "Have you experienced diarrhea or constipation?"
- **Patient**: "Yes, I've had frequent diarrhea."
- **Doctor**: "It's important to stay hydrated. Drink plenty of water."
- **Patient**: "Thank you, I will."

CULTURAL NOTES - DID YOU KNOW?

Dietary Habits and Sensitivities: Different cultures have unique dietary habits that may affect gastrointestinal health. For example, in some Latin American cultures, diets are rich in beans and spices, which could be relevant when discussing bloating or heartburn.

Traditional Remedies: Many cultures use herbal teas or home remedies for gastrointestinal issues. For instance, 'manzanilla' (chamomile tea) is commonly used in Hispanic cultures for stomach aches.

Perceptions of Digestive Health: In some cultures, digestive health is closely tied to overall well-being. Discussing gastrointestinal symptoms might require sensitivity, as patients may associate them with broader health concerns.

Communication Styles: Some cultures may be more private about discussing gastrointestinal issues. For example, talking about bowel movements may be uncomfortable for some patients, requiring a more sensitive approach.

True or False:

1. (True/False) "Hinchazón" means constipation in Spanish.
2. (True/False) "Dieta blanda" refers to a high-fiber diet.
3. (True/False) "Acidez" is the Spanish term for heartburn.

How Do You Say?

1. Avoid greasy foods

   _____

2. I have a stomach ache

   _____

3. Drink plenty of water

   _____

4. Bloating

   _____

Scenario Response:

A patient reports feeling gassy and uncomfortable after meals. What Spanish term describes this condition?

_____

COMPREHENSION RECAP ANSWERS	
True or False:	**How Do You Say?**
1. False	1. **Evite alimentos grasosos** - Avoid greasy foods
2. False	2. **Tengo dolor de estómago** - I have a stomach ache
3. True	3. **Beba mucha agua** - Drink plenty of water
	4. **Hinchazón** - Bloating

Scenario Response:

A patient reports feeling gassy and uncomfortable after meals. What Spanish term describes this condition?

Gases

Chronic Conditions

DIABETES-RELATED TERMS

1. **Glucosa** (gloo-koh-sah):

   Glucose

2. **Insulina** (een-soo-lee-nah):

   Insulin

3. **Hiperglucemia** (ee-pair-gloo-seh-mee-ah):

   Hyperglycemia

4. **Hipoglucemia** (ee-poh-gloo-seh-mee-ah):

   Hypoglycemia

5. **Automonitoreo** (ow-toh-moh-nee-toh-reh-oh):

   Self-monitoring

6. **Hemoglobina A1c** (eh-moh-gloh-bee-nah ah-oon-seh):

7. Hemoglobin A1c

8. **Bomba de insulina** (bohm-pah deh een-soo-lee-nah):

   Insulin pump

9. **Control de la dieta** (kohn-trol deh lah dee-eh-tah):

Diet control

10. **Niveles de azúcar en sangre** (nee-veh-lehs deh ah-soo-kahr ehn sahn-greh):

Blood sugar levels

11. **Administración de insulina** (ahd-mee-nees-trah-see-ohn deh een-soo-lee-nah):

Insulin administration

12. **Prueba de glucosa** (proo-eh-bah deh gloo-koh-sah):

Glucose test

13. **Plan de alimentación** (plahn deh ah-lee-men-tah-see-ohn):

Meal plan

HYPERTENSION-RELATED TERMS

1. **Presión arterial** (preh-see-ohn ahr-teh-ree-ahl):

Blood pressure

2. **Hipertensión** (ee-pair-ten-see-ohn):
Hypertension

3. **Medicamento antihipertensivo** (meh-dee-kah-men-toh ahn-tee-ee-pair-ten-see-voh): Antihypertensive medication

4. **Monitorización de la presión** (moh-nee-toh-ree-sah-see-ohn deh lah preh-see-ohn): Blood pressure monitoring

5. **Dieta baja en sal** (dee-eh-tah bah-hah ehn sahl):

   Low-salt diet

6. **Ejercicio regular** (eh-hehr-see-see-oh reh-goo-lahr):

   Regular exercise

7. **Control de peso** (kohn-trol deh peh-soh):
   Weight control

8. **Niveles de colesterol** (nee-veh-lehs deh koh-lehs-teh-rohl):

   Cholesterol levels

9. **Estrés** (ehs-trehs):

   Stress

10. **Limitar el consumo de alcohol** (lee-mee-tahr ehl kohn-soo-moh deh ahl-koh-ohl):

    Limit alcohol consumption

11. **Evitar el tabaco** (eh-vee-tahr ehl tah-bah-koh):

Avoid tobacco

_____

12. **Chequeo regular** (cheh-keh-oh reh-goo-lahr):

Regular check-up

_____

Practical Examples

1. **"Su glucosa está alta".**

(Your glucose is high.)

_____

2. **"Necesita más insulina".**

(You need more insulin.)

_____

3. **"Evite comidas con mucho azúcar".**

(Avoid foods with a lot of sugar.)

_____

4. **"Si se siente débil, coma algo dulce".**

(If you feel weak, eat something sweet.)

_____

5. **"Controle su glucosa a menudo".**

(Check your glucose often.)

_____

6. **"Anote su azúcar en sangre cada día".**

(Write down your blood sugar every day.)

_____

7. **"Mida su presión arterial todos los días".**

   (Measure your blood pressure every day.)

   _____

8. **"Coma menos sal".**

   (Eat less salt.)

   _____

9. **"Haga ejercicio regularmente".**

   (Exercise regularly.)

   _____

10. **"Siga un plan de comidas saludable".**

    (Follow a healthy meal plan.)

    _____

11. **"No beba mucho alcohol".**

    (Do not drink too much alcohol.)

    _____

12. **"Volveremos a revisar su presión".**

    (We will check your pressure again.)

    _____

Translate That Scenario!

You'll be given a simple sentence or scenario in English related to chronic conditions. Your task is to do your best to translate it into Spanish, using the words and phrases you've learned.

Scenario 1: A patient needs to adjust their insulin dosage.

_____

Scenario 2: A person is asking for dietary advice to manage high blood sugar.

_____

Scenario 3: A nurse is instructing a patient on how to monitor their blood pressure at home.

_____

Scenario 4: A doctor is explaining the importance of regular exercise for hypertension.

_____

Scenario 5: A patient is describing occasional dizziness due to low blood sugar.

_____

Scenario 1: A patient needs to adjust their insulin dosage.

Translation: "Un paciente necesita ajustar su dosis de insulina".

Scenario 2: A person is asking for dietary advice to manage high blood sugar.

Translation: "Una persona pide consejos dietéticos para manejar el azúcar alta en la sangre".

Scenario 3: A nurse is instructing a patient on how to monitor their blood pressure at home.

Translation: "Una enfermera está instruyendo a un paciente sobre cómo monitorear su presión arterial en casa".

Scenario 4: A doctor is explaining the importance of regular exercise for hypertension.

Translation: "Un médico está explicando la importancia del ejercicio regular para la hipertensión".

Scenario 5: A patient is describing occasional dizziness due to low blood sugar.

Translation: "Un paciente describe mareos ocasionales debido a su nivel bajo de azúcar en la sangre".

Dialogue 1

- **Médico**: "¿Cómo han estado sus niveles de glucosa últimamente?"
- **Paciente**: "Han estado altos. Estoy preocupado".
- **Médico**: "Necesitamos revisar y ajustar su plan de alimentación".
- **Paciente**: "Entiendo, seguiré sus recomendaciones".

Comprehension Questions:

1. What concern does the patient express about their health condition?
2. What does the doctor suggest needs to be reviewed and adjusted?
3. How does the patient respond to the doctor's suggestions?

English Translation:

- **Doctor**: "How have your glucose levels been lately?"
- **Patient**: "They have been high. I'm worried."
- **Doctor**: "We need to review and adjust your meal plan."
- **Patient**: "I understand, I'll follow your recommendations."

Dialogue 2

- **Enfermera**: "¿Está tomando su medicamento para la hipertensión regularmente?"
- **Paciente**: "Sí, todos los días. Pero, ¿debería hacer más ejercicio?"
- **Enfermera**: "Sí, el ejercicio ayuda a controlar la presión arterial".
- **Paciente**: "Voy a intentarlo. Gracias".

Comprehension Questions:

1. What is the nurse asking the patient about?
2. What additional health action does the patient inquire about?
3. What advice does the nurse give, and how does the patient respond?

English Translation:

- **Nurse**: "Are you taking your hypertension medication regularly?"
- **Patient**: "Yes, every day. But should I exercise more?"
- **Nurse**: "Yes, exercise helps control blood pressure."

◢ **Patient**: "I will try that. Thank you."

CULTURAL NOTES - DID YOU KNOW?

Dietary Preferences and Traditions: In many Hispanic cultures, traditional diets may be rich in carbohydrates and fats, which can impact diabetes management. For example, staple foods like tortillas, rice, and beans are high in carbohydrates. Understanding these dietary habits is crucial for providing realistic and culturally sensitive dietary advice.

Use of Herbal Remedies: Some patients may prefer or complement their treatment with herbal remedies or natural medicine. For instance, in Mexican culture, natural remedies like 'nopal' (prickly pear cactus) might be used to help manage blood sugar levels.

Family Involvement in Care: In many cultures, family members play a significant role in managing chronic conditions. A patient's family might be involved in monitoring dietary intake, reminding about medication, or even attending medical appointments.

Perceptions of Illness: Cultural beliefs can influence how patients perceive their illness. For instance, some may view hypertension as a temporary condition rather than a chronic one, affecting their commitment to long-term management strategies.

Language Barriers and Medical Understanding: Language barriers can sometimes lead to misunderstandings about the nature of chronic conditions and their management. Clear communication using simple, understandable terms is essential, especially when explaining complex concepts like blood glucose monitoring or the importance of regular blood pressure checks.

True or False:

1. (True/False) "Insulina" is used to treat hypertension.
2. (True/False) "Hipertensión" refers to high blood pressure.
3. (True/False) A diet high in salt is recommended for patients with hypertension.

How Do You Say?

1. Monitor your blood sugar levels daily

   _____

2. Reduce your carbohydrate intake

   _____

3. High blood pressure

   _____

4. Insulin

   _____

Scenario Response:

A patient with diabetes needs to adjust their medication. What Spanish phrase would you use to say "We need to adjust your medication"?

COMPREHENSION RECAP ANSWERS

True or False:	How Do You Say?
1. False	**1. Monitoree sus niveles de azúcar en sangre diariamente** - Monitor your blood sugar levels daily
2. True	**2. Reduzca su ingesta de carbohidratos** - Reduce your carbohydrate intake
3. False	**3. Presión arterial alta** - High blood pressure
	4. Insulina - Insulin

Scenario Response:

A patient with diabetes needs to adjust their medication. What Spanish phrase would you use to say "We need to adjust your medication"?

Necesitamos ajustar su medicamento

Cardiology

1. **Dolor de pecho** (doh-lor deh peh-choh):

   Chest pain

2. **Falta de aire** (fahl-tah deh ah-ee-reh):

   Shortness of breath

3. **Palpitaciones** (pahl-pee-tah-see-ohn-es):

   Palpitations

4. **Mareos** (mah-reh-ohs):

   Dizziness

5. **Fatiga** (fah-tee-gah):

   Fatigue

6. **Edema** (eh-deh-mah):

   Swelling

7. **Taquicardia** (tah-kee-kar-dee-ah):

   Tachycardia

8. **Arritmia** (ah-ree-t-mee-ah):

Arrhythmia

9. **Sudoración** (soo-doh-rah-see-ohn):

Sweating

10. **Desmayo** (dehs-mah-yoh):

Fainting

11. **Cianosis** (see-ah-noh-sees):

Cyanosis

12. **Angina** (ahn-hee-nah):

Angina

FAMILY HISTORY

1. **Antecedentes cardíacos** (ahn-teh-seh-den-tehs kar-dee-ah-kohs):

Cardiac history

2. **Hipertensión familiar** (ee-pair-ten-see-ohn fah-mee-lyahr):

Family history of hypertension

3. **Colesterol alto** (koh-lehs-teh-rohl ahl-toh):

High cholesterol

4. **Infarto** (een-far-toh):

Heart attack

5. **Enfermedad coronaria** (ehn-fehr-meh-dahd koh-roh-nah-ree-ah):

Coronary disease

6. **Accidente cerebrovascular** (ahk-see-den-teh seh-reh-broh-bahs-koo-lahr):

Stroke

7. **Diabetes** (dee-ah-beh-tes):

Diabetes

8. **Obesidad** (oh-beh-see-dahd):

Obesity

9. **Enfermedad vascular** (ehn-fehr-meh-dahd bahs-koo-lahr):

Vascular disease

10. **Muerte súbita** (mwer-teh soo-bee-tah):

Sudden death

11. Arritmias (ah-ree-t-mee-ahs):

Arrhythmias

12. Insuficiencia cardíaca (een-soo-fee-see-ehn-see-ah kar-dee-ah-kah):

Heart failure

LIFESTYLE FACTORS

1. Dieta (dee-eh-tah):

Diet

2. Ejercicio (eh-hehr-see-see-oh):

Exercise

3. Fumar (foo-mahr):

Smoking

4. Consumo de alcohol (kohn-soo-moh deh ahl-koh-ohl):

Alcohol consumption

5. Control de peso (kohn-trol deh peh-soh):

Weight control

6. **Manejo del estrés** (mah-neh-hoh dehl ehs-trehs):

Stress management

7. **Sueño adecuado** (swen-yoh ah-deh-kwah-doh):

Adequate sleep

8. **Alimentación saludable** (ah-lee-men-tah-see-ohn sah-loo-dah-bleh):

Healthy eating

9. **Evitar el sedentarismo** (eh-vee-tahr ehl seh-den-tah-ree-smoh):

Avoid sedentary lifestyle

10. **Controlar la hipertensión** (kohn-troh-lahr lah ee-pair-ten-see-ohn):

Control hypertension

11. **Reducir el colesterol** (reh-doo-seer ehl koh-lehs-teh-rohl):

Reduce cholesterol

12. **Monitoreo regular** (moh-nee-toh-reh-oh reh-goo-lahr):

Regular monitoring

1. **"¿Tiene dolor de pecho?"**

   (Do you have chest pain?)

   _____

2. **"Controle su colesterol".**

   (Control your cholesterol.)

   _____

3. **"Coma menos grasas".**

   (Eat less fat.)

   _____

4. **"Haga ejercicio".**

   (Exercise.)

   _____

5. **"¿Hay casos de hipertensión en su familia?"**

   (Hypertension in your family?)

   _____

6. **"Evite la obesidad".**

   (Avoid obesity.)

   _____

7. **"No fume".**

   (Do not smoke.)

   _____

8. **"Reduzca el estrés".**

   (Reduce stress.)

   _____

9. **"Duerma bien".**

(Sleep well.)

_____

10. **"No tome mucha cafeína".**

(Do not drink a lot of caffeine.)

_____

11. **"Beber alcohol moderadamente".**

(Drink alcohol moderately.)

_____

12. **"Mida su presión arterial".**

(Measure your blood pressure.)

_____

Translate That Scenario!

You'll be given a simple sentence or scenario in English related to cardiology issues. Your task is to do your best to translate it into Spanish, using the words and phrases you've learned.

Scenario 1: A patient is advised to monitor their blood pressure regularly.

_____

Scenario 2: A doctor recommends a patient to reduce salt intake for heart health.

_____

Scenario 3: A patient mentions that their family has a history of high cholesterol.

_____

Scenario 4: A nurse suggests a patient to include more exercise in their daily routine.

_____

Scenario 5: A patient complains of occasional chest pain after physical activity.

_____

Scenario 1: A patient is advised to monitor their blood pressure regularly.

Translation: "Se aconseja al paciente que monitoree su presión arterial regularmente".

Scenario 2: A doctor recommends a patient to reduce salt intake for heart health.

Translation: "Un médico recomienda al paciente reducir el consumo de sal para la salud del corazón".

Scenario 3: A patient mentions that their family has a history of high cholesterol.

Translation: "Un paciente menciona que su familia tiene antecedentes de colesterol alto".

Scenario 4: A nurse suggests a patient to include more exercise in their daily routine.

Translation: "Una enfermera sugiere al paciente incluir más ejercicio en su rutina diaria".

Scenario 5: A patient complains of occasional chest pain after physical activity.

Translation: "Un paciente se queja de dolor de pecho ocasional después de la actividad física"

Dialogue 1

- **Médico**: "¿Siente algún dolor en el pecho?"
- **Paciente**: "Sí, a veces después de caminar".
- **Médico**: "Necesitamos hacer un examen cardíaco".
- **Paciente**: "Está bien, entiendo".

Comprehension Questions:

1. What symptom does the patient report to the doctor?
2. What does the doctor decide to do next?
3. How does the patient respond to the doctor's suggestion?

English Version:

- **Doctor**: "Do you feel any chest pain?"
- **Patient**: "Yes, sometimes after walking."
- **Doctor**: "We need to do a cardiac exam."
- **Patient**: "Okay, I understand."

Dialogue 2

- **Enfermera**: "¿Ha medido su presión arterial recientemente?"
- **Paciente**: "No muy seguido. ¿Es importante?"
- **Enfermera**: "Sí, es crucial para su salud cardíaca".
- **Paciente**: "Voy a monitorearla más a menudo".

Comprehension Questions:

1. What is the nurse asking the patient about?
2. What concern does the patient express?
3. What advice does the nurse give to the patient?

English Translation:

- **Nurse**: "Have you measured your blood pressure recently?"
- **Patient**: "Not very often. Is it important?"
- **Nurse**: "Yes, it's crucial for your heart health."
- **Patient**: "I will monitor it more often."

CULTURAL NOTES - DID YOU KNOW?

Dietary Practices and Heart Health: In many Hispanic cultures, traditional diets may include foods high in saturated fats or sodium, which can impact heart health. For example, popular dishes like 'chicharrón' (fried pork skin) or 'chorizo' (spicy sausage) are high in saturated fats.

Perceptions of Exercise: Attitudes towards exercise can vary culturally. In some cultures, regular physical activity might not be as prevalent, especially in older generations. Encouraging gentle, culturally appropriate forms of exercise, like walking or traditional dancing, can be more effective.

Family History Discussions: In some cultures, discussing family health history, especially regarding conditions like heart disease or stroke, might be sensitive. It's important to approach these conversations with respect and understanding of potential cultural taboos.

Use of Traditional Remedies: Some patients may use herbal remedies or traditional practices alongside conventional medicine for heart health. For instance, herbal teas like 'té de tilo' (linden tea) are sometimes used for their perceived heart benefits.

Language and Communication Styles: It's crucial to communicate clearly and effectively, avoiding medical jargon. In some cultures, direct communication about serious health issues like heart disease might be less common, requiring a more nuanced approach.

Stress and Heart Health: Different cultures may have various ways of dealing with stress, which is an important factor in heart health. Understanding these coping mechanisms can help in providing holistic care.

True or False:

1. (True/False) "Palpitaciones" can be a symptom of heart problems.
2. (True/False) "Edema" is related to brain health, not heart health.
3. (True/False) Regular exercise is important for maintaining heart health.

How Do You Say?

1. Avoid high cholesterol foods

   _____

2. I need to measure my blood pressure

   _____

3. Heart attack

   _____

4. Family history of heart disease

   _____

Scenario Response:

A patient reports feeling dizzy and having chest pain after exercise. What Spanish term would describe their condition?

_____

COMPREHENSION RECAP ANSWERS	
True or False:	**How Do You Say?**
1. True 2. False 3. True	1. **Evite alimentos con alto colesterol** – Avoid high cholesterol foods 2. **Necesito medir mi presión arterial** – I need to measure my blood pressure 3. **Infarto** – Heart attach 4. **Historial familiar de enfermedades cardíacas** – Family history of heart disease

Scenario Response:

A patient reports feeling dizzy and having chest pain after exercise. What Spanish term would describe their condition?

Mareos y dolor de pecho después del ejercicio.

Mental Health

MENTAL HEALTH SYMPTOMS

1. **Ansiedad** (ahn-see-eh-dahd):

   Anxiety

2. **Depresión** (deh-preh-see-ohn):

   Depression

3. **Estrés** (ehs-trehs):

   Stress

4. **Insomnio** (een-sohm-nee-oh):

   Insomnia

5. **Fatiga** (fah-tee-gah):

   Fatigue

6. **Cambios de humor** (kahm-byohs deh ooh-mor):

   Mood swings

7. **Pánico** (pah-nee-koh):

   Panic

8. **Fobia** (foh-bee-ah):

Phobia

9. **Obsesiones** (ohb-seh-see-oh-nehs):

Obsessions

10. **Compulsiones** (kohm-pool-see-oh-nehs):

Compulsions

11. **Tristeza** (trees-tay-sah):

Sadness

12. **Irritabilidad** (ee-ree-tah-bee-lee-dahd):

Irritability

TREATMENT OPTIONS

1. **Terapia** (teh-rah-pee-ah):

Therapy

2. **Medicamento** (meh-dee-kah-men-toh):

Medication

3. **Consejería** (kohn-seh-heh-ree-ah):

Counseling

4. **Meditación** (meh-dee-tah-see-ohn):

Meditation

5. **Psicoterapia** (see-koh-teh-rah-pee-ah):

Psychotherapy

6. **Tratamiento cognitivo-conductual**

(trah-tah-mee-en-toh kohg-nee-tee-voh-kohn-dook-too-ahl):

Cognitive-behavioral therapy

7. **Antidepresivos** (ahn-tee-deh-preh-see-vohs):

Antidepressants

8. **Ansiolíticos** (ahn-see-oh-lee-tee-kohs):

Anxiolytics

9. **Hospitalización** (oh-spee-tah-lee-sah-see-ohn):

Hospitalization

10. **Apoyo grupal** (ah-poh-yoh groo-pahl):

Group support

11. **Terapia de relajación** (teh-rah-pee-ah deh reh-lah-hah-see-ohn):

Relaxation therapy

12. **Manejo del estrés** (mah-neh-hoh dehl ehs-trehs):

Stress management

SUPPORT MECHANISMS

1. **Apoyo familiar** (ah-poh-yoh fah-mee-lyahr):

Family support

2. **Redes sociales** (reh-dehs soh-see-ah-lehs):

Social networks

3. **Grupos de apoyo** (groo-pohs deh ah-poh-yoh):

Support groups

4. **Actividades recreativas** (ahk-tee-vee-dah-dehs reh-kreh-ah-tee-vahs):

Recreational activities

5. **Ejercicio físico** (eh-hehr-see-see-oh fees-ee-koh):

Physical exercise

6. **Dieta equilibrada** (dee-eh-tah eh-kee-lee-brah-dah):

   Balanced diet

7. **Tiempo de ocio** (tyehm-poh deh oh-see-oh):

   Leisure time

8. **Escritura terapéutica** (eh-skree-too-rah teh-rah-peh-oo-tee-kah):

   Therapeutic writing

9. **Arte terapia** (ahr-teh teh-rah-pee-ah):

   Art therapy

10. **Voluntariado** (voh-loon-tah-ree-ah-doh):

    Volunteering

11. **Yoga** (yoh-gah):

    Yoga

12. **Respiración consciente** (rehs-pee-rah-see-ohn kohn-see-ehn-teh):

    Mindful breathing

Practical Examples

1. **"¿Siente ansiedad o estrés?"**

   (Do you feel anxiety or stress?)

2. **"Considere terapia para la depresión".**

   (Consider therapy for depression.)

3. **"La meditación reduce el estrés".**

   (Meditation reduces stress.)

4. **"Tome medicamento para la ansiedad".**

   (Take medication for anxiety.)

5. **"La terapia cognitiva es útil".**

   (Cognitive therapy is useful.)

6. **"El apoyo de la familia ayuda".**

   (Support from family helps.)

7. **"Los grupos de apoyo son buenos".**

   (Support groups are good.)

8. **"Haga ejercicio para su bienestar mental".**

   (Exercise for mental well-being.)

9. **"Una dieta sana mejora el ánimo".**

   (A healthy diet improves mood.)

   _____

10. **"Use respiración consciente para calmarse".**

    (Use mindful breathing to calm.)

    _____

11. **"Escribir sus pensamientos ayuda".**

    (Writing your thoughts helps.)

    _____

12. **"El yoga ayuda con el estrés".**

    (Yoga helps with stress.)

    _____

Translate That Scenario!

You'll be given a simple sentence or scenario in English related to mental health issues. Your task is to do your best to translate it into Spanish, using the words and phrases you've learned.

Scenario 1: A patient mentions they have been feeling very anxious lately.

_____

Scenario 2: A doctor advises a patient to try meditation for stress relief.

_____

Scenario 3: A patient is asked about their family's history of depression.

_____

Scenario 4: A nurse suggests joining a support group for emotional well-being.

_____

Scenario 5: A patient is looking for ways to improve their mood through diet.

_____

Scenario 1: A patient mentions they have been feeling very anxious lately.

Translation: "Un paciente menciona que se ha sentido muy ansioso últimamente".

Scenario 2: A doctor advises a patient to try meditation for stress relief.

Translation: "Un médico aconseja al paciente probar la meditación para aliviar el estrés".

Scenario 3: A patient is asked about their family's history of depression.

Translation: "Se le pregunta al paciente sobre antecedentes de depresión en su familia".

Scenario 4: A nurse suggests joining a support group for emotional well-being.

Translation: "Una enfermera sugiere unirse a un grupo de apoyo para el bienestar emocional".

Scenario 5: A patient is looking for ways to improve their mood through diet.

Translation: "Un paciente busca formas de mejorar su ánimo a través de la dieta".

Dialogue 1

- **Médico**: "¿Ha sentido ansiedad últimamente?"
- **Paciente**: "Sí, me siento ansioso a menudo".
- **Médico**: "Recomiendo la meditación para ayudar a reducir la ansiedad".
- **Paciente**: "Lo intentaré, gracias".

Comprehension Questions:

1. What symptom is the patient experiencing?
2. What does the doctor recommend to help reduce it?
3. How does the patient respond to the doctor's recommendation?

English Version:

- **Doctor:** "Have you felt anxious lately?"
- **Patient**: "Yes, I often feel anxious."
- **Doctor**: "I recommend meditation to help reduce anxiety."
- **Patient**: "I will try that, thank you."

Dialogue 2

- **Enfermera**: "¿Cómo ha sido su estado de ánimo recientemente?"
- **Paciente**: "He estado un poco deprimido".
- **Enfermera**: "Unirse a un grupo de apoyo puede ser beneficioso".
- **Paciente**: "Eso suena bien. Buscaré uno".

Comprehension Questions:

1. What mental health issue does the patient mention?
2. What suggestion does the nurse make for the patient?
3. What is the patient's reaction to the nurse's suggestion?

English Translation:

- **Nurse**: "How has your mood been recently?"
- **Patient**: "I have been a bit depressed."
- **Nurse**: "Joining a support group can be beneficial."
- **Patient**: "That sounds good. I'll look for one."

CULTURAL NOTES - DID YOU KNOW?

Stigma in Mental Health: Stigma, especially prevalent in some cultures like Hispanic communities, leads to reluctance in discussing or seeking help for mental health issues due to fear of judgment.

Family's Role and Cultural Expression: Family dynamics significantly influence mental health in many cultures. Additionally, psychological distress might be expressed through physical symptoms, which is important to recognize for accurate diagnosis.

Traditional Healing and Communication: Respect for traditional healing methods, like those in Latin American cultures, and adapting communication styles, such as using metaphors, are key in sensitive mental health discussions.

Religion and Immigrant Experiences: Religion and spirituality often play a vital role in mental health. Additionally, understanding the unique challenges faced by immigrants, such as cultural adaptation, is crucial for providing empathetic care.

These cultural insights are not just about understanding different backgrounds; they're about connecting with patients on a deeper level, offering support that acknowledges and respects their unique experiences and perspectives.

True or False:

1. (True/False) "Ansiedad" means depression.
2. (True/False) Meditation can be beneficial for stress management.
3. (True/False) "Apoyo familiar" refers to medication treatment.

How Do You Say?

1. I feel stressed and anxious

   _____

2. Joining a support group can help

   _____

3. Mood swings

   _____

4. Therapy

   _____

Scenario Response:

A patient describes feeling continuously sad and losing interest in daily activities. What Spanish term would you use to describe their condition?

_____

COMPREHENSION RECAP ANSWERS	
True or False:	**How Do You Say?**
1. False 2. True 3. False	1. **Me siento estresado y ansioso** - I feel stressed and anxious 2. **Unirse a un grupo de apoyo puede ayudar** - Joining a support group can help 3. **Cambios de humor** - Mood swings 4. **Terapia** - Therapy

Scenario Response:

A patient describes feeling continuously sad and losing interest in daily activities. What Spanish term would you use to describe their condition?

Depresión

Comfort and Instructions

COMFORTING PHRASES

1. **Tranquilo/a** (trahn-kee-loh/ah):

   Calm down

2. **Está bien** (ehs-tah byen):

   It's okay

3. **No se preocupe** (noh seh preh-oh-koo-peh):

   Don't worry

4. **Va a mejorar** (vah ah meh-hoh-rahr):

   It will get better

5. **Estoy aquí para ayudar** (ehs-toy ah-kee pah-rah ah-yoo-dahr):

   I'm here to help

6. **Respire profundamente** (reh-spee-reh proh-foon-dah-men-teh):

   Breathe deeply

7. **Estamos cuidando de usted** (ehs-tah-mohs kwee-dahn-doh deh oo-stehd):

   We're taking care of you

8. **Relájese** (reh-lah-heh-seh):

   Relax

9. **Cuénteme más** (kwehn-teh-meh mahs):

   Tell me more

10. **Lo/la entiendo** (loh/lah ehn-tyehn-doh):

    I understand you

11. **Es normal sentirse así** (ehs nohr-mahl sehn-teer-seh ah-see):

    It's normal to feel this way

12. **Vamos a ayudarle** (vah-mohs ah ah-yoo-dahr-leh):

    We are going to help you

PATIENT INSTRUCTIONS

1. **Tome este medicamento** (toh-meh ehs-teh meh-dee-kah-men-toh):

   Take this medication

2. **Descanse** (dehs-kahn-seh):

   Rest

3. **Vuelva para una revisión** (vwehl-vah pah-rah oon-ah reh-vee-see-ohn):

   Come back for a check-up

4. **Siga estas indicaciones** (see-gah ehs-tahs een-dee-kah-see-oh-nehs):

   Follow these instructions

5. **Haga estos ejercicios** (ah-gah ehs-tohs eh-hehr-see-see-ohs):

   Do these exercises

6. **Coma saludable** (koh-mah sah-loo-dah-bleh):

   Eat healthily

7. **Beba mucha agua** (beh-bah moo-chah ah-gwah):

   Drink plenty of water

8. **Evite el estrés** (eh-vee-teh ehl ehs-trehs):

   Avoid stress

9. **No levante objetos pesados** (noh leh-vahn-teh ohb-heh-tohs peh-sah-dohs):

   Don't lift heavy objects

10. **Monitoree su presión arterial** (moh-nee-toh-reh-eh soo preh-see-ohn ahr-teh-ree-ahl):

    Monitor your blood pressure

11. **Cambie el vendaje diariamente** (kahm-byeh ehl vehn-dah-heh dee-ah-ree-ah-men-teh):

Change the dressing daily

_____

12. **Use muletas** (oo-seh moo-leh-tahs):

Use crutches

Practical Examples

1. **"Tranquilo/a, estamos aquí para ayudarle".**

   (Calm down, we are here to help you.)

2. **"Tome este medicamento con agua".**

   (Take this medication with water.)

3. **"Descanse y evite actividades físicas intensas".**

   (Rest and avoid intense physical activities.)

4. **"Respire profundamente para relajarse".**

   (Breathe deeply to relax.)

5. **"Vuelva la próxima semana para una revisión".**

   (Come back next week for a check-up.)

6. **"Siga las indicaciones para su recuperación".**

   (Follow the instructions for your recovery.)

   _____

7. **"Haga estos ejercicios para mejorar".**

   (Do these exercises to improve.)

   _____

8. **"Coma alimentos saludables para sentirse mejor".**

   (Eat healthy foods to feel better.)

   _____

9. **"Beba mucha agua durante el día".**

   (Drink plenty of water throughout the day.)

   _____

10. **"Evite levantar objetos pesados por ahora".**

    (Avoid lifting heavy objects for now.)

    _____

11. **"Monitoree su presión arterial regularmente".**

    (Monitor your blood pressure regularly.)

    _____

12. **"Cámbiese el vendaje diariamente para evitar infecciones".**

    (Change the dressing daily to avoid infections.)

    _____

Translate That Scenario!

You'll be given a simple sentence or scenario in English related to comfort and instructions. Your task is to do your best to translate it into Spanish, using the words and phrases you've learned.

Scenario 1: A nurse instructs a patient to take their medication three times a day.

_____

Scenario 2: A doctor advises a patient to rest and avoid heavy lifting after surgery.

_____

Scenario 3: A healthcare provider tells a patient to come back in two weeks for a follow-up.

_____

Scenario 4: A patient is instructed to do light exercises to aid their recovery.

_____

Scenario 5: A nurse tells a patient to drink more water to stay hydrated.

_____

Scenario 1: A nurse instructs a patient to take their medication three times a day.

Translation: "Una enfermera le indica al paciente tomar su medicamento tres veces al día".

Scenario 2: A doctor advises a patient to rest and avoid heavy lifting after surgery.

Translation: "Un médico aconseja al paciente descansar y evitar levantar objetos pesados después de la cirugía".

Scenario 3: A healthcare provider tells a patient to come back in two weeks for a follow-up.

Translation: "Un profesional de la salud le dice al paciente que vuelva en dos semanas para un seguimiento".

Scenario 4: A patient is instructed to do light exercises to aid their recovery.

Translation: "Se le indica al paciente hacer ejercicios ligeros para ayudar en su recuperación".

Scenario 5: A nurse tells a patient to drink more water to stay hydrated.

Translation: "Una enfermera le dice al paciente que beba más agua para mantenerse hidratado".

Dialogue 1

- **Médico:** "Tranquilo, estamos aquí para ayudarle. ¿Cómo se ha sentido últimamente?"
- **Paciente**: "No muy bien. He tenido mucho estrés".
- **Médico**: "Respire profundamente y trate de relajarse. Evite el estrés y descanse más".
- **Paciente**: "Gracias, seguiré sus consejos".

Comprehension Questions:

1. What comforting phrase does the doctor use to reassure the patient?
2. What issue is the patient experiencing?
3. What advice does the doctor give to the patient?

English Translation:

- **Doctor**: "Calm down, we are here to help you. How have you been feeling lately?"
- **Patient**: "Not very well. I've been very stressed."
- **Doctor**: "Breathe deeply and try to relax. Avoid stress and rest more."
- **Patient**: "Thank you, I will follow your advice."

Dialogue 2

- **Enfermera:** "¿Ha seguido las indicaciones que le dimos?"
- **Paciente:** "Sí, he cambiado el vendaje diariamente y he descansado mucho".
- **Enfermera:** "Excelente. Recuerde comer saludable y beber mucha agua".
- **Paciente:** "Lo haré. Gracias por cuidarme".

Comprehension Questions:

1. What does the nurse ask the patient about?
2. What has the patient been doing as part of their care?
3. What additional advice does the nurse give?

English Translation:

- ◢ **Nurse:** "Have you followed the instructions we gave you?"
- ◢ **Patient:** "Yes, I have changed the dressing daily and rested a lot."
- ◢ **Nurse:** "Excellent. Remember to eat healthily and drink plenty of water."
- ◢ **Patient:** "I will. Thank you for taking care of me."

CULTURAL NOTES - DID YOU KNOW?

Communication Styles: Be aware that some patients may not openly express discomfort due to cultural norms of resilience. Observing non-verbal cues becomes crucial.

Family Involvement: In many cultures, family plays a critical role in patient care. Ensure to include them in discussions and care plans whenever appropriate.

Clear Instructions: Use simple, non-medical language for instructions, especially important for those with limited health literacy or non-native English speakers.

Cultural Views on Recovery: Recovery perceptions vary across cultures. Balance rest and activity recommendations according to the patient's cultural background.

Dietary Advice: Respect cultural dietary habits when suggesting changes. Food holds significant cultural value.

Alternative Remedies: Acknowledge the use of traditional remedies in many cultures. These can often complement conventional care.

Respect for Elders: Extra respect and patience are key when dealing with elderly patients, as many cultures place high value on age and experience.

Physical Contact: Understand the cultural norms around physical touch; it can be a source of comfort for some and discomfort for others.

Comprehension Recap

True or False:

1. (True/False) "Tranquilo/a" is a phrase used to calm a patient.
2. (True/False) "Descanse" means to exercise.
3. (True/False) "Tome este medicamento con agua" translates to "Take this medicine with water."

How Do You Say?

1. You need to rest for a few days

   _____

2. Please follow these instructions carefully

   _____

3. Drink plenty of water

   _____

4. Breath deeply

   _____

Scenario Response:

A patient appears anxious and is breathing rapidly. What Spanish phrase would you use to instruct them to calm down and breathe slowly?

_____

COMPREHENSION RECAP ANSWERS

True or False:	How Do You Say?
1. True	1. **Necesita descansar unos días.** - You need to rest for a few days
2. False	2. **Por favor, siga estas instrucciones cuidadosamente.** - Please follow these instructions carefully
3. True	3. **Beba mucha agua.** - Drink plenty of water
	4. **Respire profundamente.** - Breathe deeply

Scenario Response:

A patient appears anxious and is breathing rapidly. What Spanish phrase would you use to instruct them to calm down and breathe slowly?

Tranquilo/a, respire lento y profundo.

50 REAL-LIFE MEDICAL SPANISH DIALOGUES TO HELP YOU COMMUNICATE EFFECTIVELY

In this unit, you'll step into the shoes of a healthcare professional navigating a diverse range of medical encounters. From the immediacy of emergency care to the nuances of chronic condition management, these dialogues are designed to enhance your Spanish proficiency while deepening your understanding of the patient experience.

As you progress, you'll find that empathy and clarity are the heartbeat of every conversation. The dialogues are infused with real patient expressions, helping you grasp not just the language, but also the human element of healthcare. You'll learn to mirror this empathy in your responses, ensuring your communication is both medically accurate and emotionally attuned.

Now we begin the journey to strengthen your professional skills with a blend of linguistic precision, cultural sensitivity, and heartfelt empathy. Let's bridge language gaps and elevate patient care together.

Emergency Situations: Immediate care, Symptoms, and Urgency

Effective communication is vital in any emergency. This series will guide you through Spanish dialogues crucial for immediate care situations. You'll learn to articulate symptoms with precision, ask the right questions during chest pain assessments, and respond to urgent cases like severe allergic reactions and fractures. These dialogues are crafted to help you convey urgency and provide clear instructions when every second counts.

Diálogo 1:

Dolor de pecho - Chest Pain

Médico: Buenos días, ¿cómo puedo ayudarlo?

Paciente: Hola, tengo un dolor fuerte en el pecho y me cuesta respirar. Estoy un poco asustado.

Médico: Entiendo su preocupación. ¿Ha tenido este tipo de dolor antes?

Paciente: No, nunca. Empezó hace una hora y no sé qué hacer.

Médico: Mantengamos la calma. Voy a revisar su presión arterial y su corazón ahora mismo. ¿Tiene antecedentes de problemas cardíacos en su familia?

Paciente: Sí, mi padre tuvo un infarto. ¿Cree que me está pasando lo mismo?

Médico: Estamos aquí para averiguarlo y cuidar de usted. Necesitamos hacerle un electrocardiograma y análisis de sangre inmediatamente para entender mejor su situación.

Paciente: Está bien, gracias por su ayuda y por explicarme todo.

Preguntas de comprensión:

1. **¿Qué le duele al paciente?**
   a. La cabeza
   b. El brazo
   c. El pecho
   d. La espalda

2. **¿Qué antecedente familiar menciona el paciente?**
   a. Diabetes
   b. Infarto
   c. Hipertensión
   d. Artritis

3. **¿Qué procedimiento médico sugiere el doctor?**
   a. Una resonancia magnética
   b. Un electrocardiograma
   c. Una radiografía
   d. Un ultrasonido

Dialogue 1:

Chest Pain - Dolor de pecho

Doctor: "Good morning, how can I help you?"

Patient: "Hello, I have severe chest pain and I'm having trouble breathing. I'm a bit scared."

Doctor: "I understand your concern. Have you had this type of pain before?"

Patient: "No, never. It started an hour ago and I don't know what to do."

Doctor: "Let's stay calm together. I'm going to check your blood pressure and heart right now. Do you have a history of heart problems in your family?"

Patient: "Yes, my father had a heart attack. Do you think the same thing is happening to me?"

Doctor: "We're here to find out and take care of you. We need to do an electrocardiogram and a blood test immediately to better understand your situation."

Patient: "Okay, thank you for helping me and for explaining everything."

Comprehension Questions

1. **What is causing the patient pain?**
   a. Head
   b. Arm
   c. Chest
   d. Back

2. **What family history does the patient mention?**
   a. Diabetes
   b. Heart attack
   c. Hypertension
   d. Arthritis

3. **What medical procedure does the doctor suggest?**
   a. An MRI
   b. An electrocardiogram
   c. An X-ray
   d. An ultrasound

Answers

1. **c)** El pecho - Chest
2. **b)** Infarto - Heart attack
3. **b)** Un electrocardiograma - An electrocardiogram

Reacción alérgica grave - Severe Allergic Reaction

Doctor: Intenta tranquilizarte y cuéntame, ¿cómo te sientes?

Paciente: Me siento mareado y no puedo respirar bien. Tengo mucho miedo.

Doctor: Entiendo tu preocupación y estamos aquí para ayudarte. ¿Has tenido alergias anteriormente?

Paciente: Sí, soy alérgico a los frutos secos. ¿Cree que sea una reacción alérgica?

Doctor: Parece probable. Vamos a administrarte un tratamiento de inmediato para ayudarte.

Paciente: ¿Qué tratamiento recibiré?

Doctor: Te daremos un antihistamínico y epinefrina. Estos medicamentos ayudarán a aliviar tu dificultad para respirar y el mareo.

Paciente: ¿Y eso hará que me sienta mejor rápido?

Doctor: Sí, estos medicamentos actúan rápido. Te cuidaremos y monitorearemos de cerca tu mejoría.

Preguntas de comprensión

1. **¿Cuál es el síntoma principal que menciona el paciente?**
   a. Dolor de cabeza
   b. Mareo y dificultad para respirar
   c. Fiebre
   d. Náuseas

2. **¿A qué es alérgico el paciente?**
   a. Lácteos
   b. Mariscos
   c. Frutos secos
   d. Gluten

3. **¿Qué tratamiento propone el doctor?**
   a. Antibióticos
   b. Antihistamínico y epinefrina
   c. Paracetamol
   d. Reposo absoluto

Dialogue 2:

Severe Allergic Reaction - Reacción alérgica grave

Doctor: Take a moment and tell me, how are you feeling?

Patient: I feel dizzy and it's hard to breathe. I'm really scared.

Doctor: I understand your worry, and we're here to help you. Have you had allergies in the past?

Patient: Yes, I'm allergic to nuts. Do you think this is an allergic reaction?

Doctor: It seems likely. We're going to give you treatment right away to help you.

Patient: What treatment will I receive?

Doctor: We'll administer an antihistamine and epinephrine. These medications will help relieve your breathing difficulty and dizziness.

Patient: Will that make me feel better quickly?

Doctor: Yes, these medications work fast. We'll take care of you and monitor your improvement closely.

Comprehension Questions

1. **What is the main symptom mentioned by the patient?**
   a. Headache
   b. Dizziness and difficulty breathing
   c. Fever
   d. Nausea

2. **What is the patient allergic to?**
   a. Dairy
   b. Seafood
   c. Nuts
   d. Gluten

3. **What treatment does the doctor propose?**
   a. Antibiotics
   b. Antihistamine and epinephrine
   c. Paracetamol
   d. Complete rest

Answers

1. **b)** Mareo y dificultad para respirar - Dizziness and difficulty breathing
2. **c)** Frutos secos - Nuts
3. **b)** Antihistamínico y epinefrina - Antihistamine and epinephrine

Doctor: Intenta tranquilizarte y cuéntame qué te sucedió.

Paciente: Doctor, me caí por las escaleras y creo que me rompí el brazo. Me duele muchísimo y no puedo moverlo.

Doctor: Lamento mucho que estés pasando por esto. Vamos a hacerte una radiografía para ver exactamente qué ha ocurrido. Muéstrame dónde sientes más dolor.

Paciente: Aquí, en esta zona cerca de la muñeca. Y mi brazo se ve torcido.

Doctor: Entiendo, parece ser una fractura. Lo primero es aliviar tu dolor, y después vamos a colocarte una férula para mantener el brazo inmovilizado.

Paciente: ¿Así me aliviaré más rápido? ¿Cuánto tiempo tomará recuperarme?

Doctor: La férula ayuda a que los huesos se reparen adecuadamente, y ese proceso suele tomar de seis a ocho semanas. Te daremos todas las indicaciones necesarias para el cuidado en casa.

Preguntas de comprensión

1. **¿Qué le pasó al paciente?**
   a. Se cortó
   b. Se cayó
   c. Se quemó
   d. Se golpeó la cabeza

2. **¿Qué parte del cuerpo se lesionó el paciente?**
   a. La pierna
   b. El tobillo
   c. El brazo
   d. La espalda

3. **¿Cuál es el tratamiento inmediato que propone el doctor?**
   a. Poner una inyección
   b. Colocar una férula
   c. Tomar antibióticos
   d. Realizar una cirugía

Dialogue 3:
Broken Limb - Fractura ósea

Doctor: Take your time and tell me what happened.

Patient: Doctor, I fell down the stairs and I think my arm is broken. It's very painful and I can't move it.

Doctor: I'm very sorry you're going through this. We're going to do an X-ray to see exactly what's going on. Show me where you're feeling the most pain.

Patient: Right here, near the wrist. Also, my arm looks bent.

Doctor: I see, it does look like a fracture. Our first step is to relieve your pain, and then we'll apply a splint to keep your arm immobilized.

Patient: Will that help it heal faster? How long is the recovery going to take?

Doctor: The splint ensures your bone heals properly. Healing usually takes six to eight weeks. We will provide you with all the necessary instructions for your care at home.

Comprehension Questions

1. **What happened to the patient?**
   a. Got a cut
   b. Fell down
   c. Got burned
   d. Hit their head

2. **Which part of the body did the patient injure?**
   a. The leg
   b. The ankle
   c. The arm
   d. The back

3. **What is the immediate treatment the doctor proposes?**
   a. Give an injection
   b. Apply a splint
   c. Take antibiotics
   d. Perform surgery

Answers

1. **b)** Se cayó - Fell down
2. **c)** El brazo - The arm
3. **b)** Colocar una férula - Apply a splint

Diálogo 4:
Crisis asmática - Asthma Attack

Doctor: ¿Cómo se siente? Cuénteme con detalle.

Paciente: No puedo respirar bien y siento mi pecho muy apretado. Estoy muy preocupado.

Doctor: Entiendo su preocupación. ¿Usted tiene asma?

Paciente: Sí, soy asmático y olvidé mi inhalador en casa. ¿Qué puedo hacer ahora?

Doctor: Le vamos a administrar un broncodilatador ahora mismo para ayudarle a respirar. ¿Recuerda cuándo comenzaron estos síntomas?

Paciente: Empezaron hace unos minutos, después de subir unas escaleras. Me falta el aire.

Doctor: Le entiendo, lo importante es que intente mantenerse tranquilo. Vamos a monitorear su respiración y el oxígeno en su sangre para asegurarnos de que mejora.

Preguntas de comprensión

1. **¿Qué síntoma principal tiene el paciente?**
   a. Dolor de cabeza
   b. Dificultad para respirar
   c. Dolor de estómago
   d. Fiebre

2. **¿Qué olvidó el paciente?**
   a. Su medicamento
   b. Su inhalador
   c. Su cita médica
   d. Su identificación

3. **¿Qué le da el doctor al paciente?**
   a. Un analgésico
   b. Un antibiótico
   c. Un broncodilatador
   d. Una vacuna

Dialogue 4:
Asthma Attack - Crisis asmática

Doctor: How do you feel? Please, tell me in detail.

Patient: I'm having trouble breathing and my chest feels really tight. I'm quite worried.

Doctor: I understand your concern. Do you have asthma?

Patient: Yes, I'm asthmatic and I forgot my inhaler at home. What can I do now?

Doctor: We're going to administer a bronchodilator right now to help you breathe. Do you remember when these symptoms started?

Patient: They started a few minutes ago, after climbing some stairs. I'm feeling very breathless.

Doctor: I understand, the important thing is to try and stay calm. We're going to monitor your breathing and blood oxygen to make sure you improve.

Comprehension Questions

1. **What is the main symptom the patient is experiencing?**
   a. Headache
   b. Difficulty breathing
   c. Stomach pain
   d. Fever

2. **What did the patient forget?**
   a. Their medication
   b. Their inhaler
   c. Their medical appointment
   d. Their identification

3. **What does the doctor give to the patient?**
   a. A painkiller
   b. An antibiotic
   c. A bronchodilator
   d. A vaccine

Answers

1. **b)** Dificultad para respirar - Difficulty breathing
2. **b)** Su inhalador - Their inhaler
3. **c)** Un broncodilatador - A bronchodilator

Diálogo 5:

Quemadura grave - Severe Burn

Doctor: ¿Qué le sucedió? Cuénteme con calma.

Paciente: Me quemé con aceite hirviendo mientras cocinaba. Fue un accidente y me duele mucho.

Doctor: Veo que está preocupado. Vamos a ver qué parte del cuerpo se quemó.

Paciente: Es mi mano y parte del brazo. La piel está muy roja y tiene ampollas.

Doctor: Lo primero es enfriar la quemadura y luego aplicaremos un vendaje especial. ¿Ha tomado algún analgésico?

Paciente: No, no he tomado nada. ¿Qué puedo hacer para el dolor?

Doctor: Le vamos a dar algo para el dolor y para prevenir infecciones. Es importante que regrese para una revisión y un cambio de vendaje.

Preguntas de comprensión

1. **¿Cómo se quemó el paciente?**
   a. Con fuego
   b. Con aceite hirviendo
   c. Con agua caliente
   d. Con un objeto caliente

2. **¿Qué partes del cuerpo se quemaron?**
   a. La cara y el cuello
   b. La mano y el brazo
   c. La pierna y el pie
   d. La espalda

3. **¿Cuál es el tratamiento inmediato para la quemadura?**
   a. Aplicar hielo
   b. Tomar un antihistamínico
   c. Usar una crema antibiótica
   d. Enfriar y vendar

Dialogue 5:

Severe Burn - Quemadura grave

Doctor: What happened to you? Please, tell me calmly.

Patient: I got burned with boiling oil while cooking. It was an accident, and it hurts a lot.

Doctor: I see that you're worried. Let's see which part of the body got burned.

Patient: It's my hand and part of my arm. The skin is very red and blistered.

Doctor: First, we'll cool the burn, then we'll apply a special dressing. Have you taken any painkillers?

Patient: No, I haven't taken anything. What can I do for the pain?

Doctor: We will give you something for the pain and to prevent infection. It's important for you to come back for a check-up and dressing change.

Comprehension Questions

1. **How did the patient get burned?**
   - a. Fire
   - b. Boiling oil
   - c. Hot water
   - d. A hot object

2. **Which parts of the body did the burn affect?**
   - a. The face and neck
   - b. The hand and arm
   - c. The leg and foot
   - d. The back

3. **What is the immediate treatment for the burn?**
   - a. Apply ice
   - b. Take an antihistamine
   - c. Use an antibiotic cream
   - d. Cool and dress

Answers

1. **b)** Con aceite hirviendo - With boiling oil
2. **b)** La mano y el brazo - The hand and arm
3. **d)** Enfriar y vendar - Cool and dress

Lesión en la cabeza - Head Injury

Paciente: Doctor, me golpeé la cabeza al caer de una escalera. Ahora me siento mareado y un poco aturdido.

Doctor: Cuénteme más sobre la caída. ¿En algún momento perdió el conocimiento?

Paciente: No, no perdí el conocimiento, pero el dolor es intenso y siento náuseas.

Doctor: Entiendo. Vamos a revisarlo cuidadosamente. Es importante descartar una conmoción cerebral. Trate de mantenerse despierto y quieto.

Paciente: ¿Cree que necesitaré una radiografía o algo más?

Doctor: Sí, haremos una radiografía y posiblemente una tomografía computarizada para verificar que no haya lesiones internas. Vamos a cuidar bien de usted.

Preguntas de comprensión

1. **¿Qué le pasó al paciente?**
   a. Se cortó en la cabeza
   b. Se golpeó la cabeza
   c. Se quemó la cabeza
   d. Se picó la cabeza

2. **¿Cuáles son los síntomas del paciente después del golpe?**
   a. Pérdida de conciencia y sangrado
   b. Visión borrosa y fiebre
   c. Dolor de cabeza y náuseas
   d. Confusión y pérdida de audición

3. **¿Qué pruebas sugiere el doctor?**
   a. Un electroencefalograma
   b. Una radiografía y una tomografía
   c. Análisis de sangre
   d. Una resonancia magnética

Dialogue 6:
Head Injury - Lesión en la cabeza

Patient: Doctor, I hit my head when I fell off a ladder. Now, I feel dizzy and a bit confused.

Doctor: Tell me more about the fall. Did you lose consciousness at any point?

Patient: No, I didn't lose consciousness, but the pain is intense, and I feel nauseous.

Doctor: I see. We're going to examine you thoroughly. It's important to rule out a concussion. Try to stay awake and still.

Patient: Do you think I will need an X-ray or something more?

Doctor: Yes, we'll do an X-ray and possibly a CT scan to make sure there are no internal injuries. We will take good care of you.

Comprehension Questions

1. **What happened to the patient?**
   a. Cut his head
   b. Hit his head
   c. Burned his head
   d. Stung his head

2. **What are the patient's symptoms after the injury?**
   a. Loss of consciousness and bleeding
   b. Blurred vision and fever
   c. Headache and nausea
   d. Confusion and hearing loss

3. **What tests does the doctor suggest?**
   a. An electroencephalogram
   b. An X-ray and a CT scan
   c. Blood tests
   d. An MRI

Answers

1. **b)** Se golpeó la cabeza - Hit his head
2. **c)** Dolor de cabeza y náuseas - Headache and nausea
3. **b)** Una radiografía y una tomografía - An X-ray and a CT scan

Diálogo 7:
Envenenamiento - Poisoning

Paciente: Doctor, creo que sin querer ingerí algo tóxico.

Doctor: Mantengamos la calma. Cuéntame, ¿qué crees que has ingerido?

Paciente: No estoy seguro, pero había un producto de limpieza abierto en la cocina.

Doctor: Entiendo tu preocupación, y vamos a ayudarte. ¿Tienes náuseas, vómitos o mareos?

Paciente: Sí, y tengo un dolor fuerte en el estómago.

Doctor: Actuaremos de inmediato para ayudarte. Vamos a realizar un lavado gástrico y unos análisis para ver qué ha sucedido. No te preocupes, estás en buenas manos y vamos a cuidarte.

Preguntas de comprensión

1. **¿Qué cree el paciente que ha ingerido?**
   a. Medicamentos caducados
   b. Alimentos en mal estado
   c. Una sustancia tóxica
   d. Alcohol en exceso

2. **¿Dónde encontró el paciente la sustancia sospechosa?**
   a. En el baño
   b. En la cocina
   c. En el jardín
   d. En el garaje

3. **¿Qué procedimiento médico menciona el doctor?**
   a. Una transfusión de sangre
   b. Un lavado gástrico
   c. Una resonancia magnética
   d. Un electrocardiograma

Dialogue 7:
Poisoning - Envenenamiento

Patient: Doctor, I think I may have accidentally ingested something toxic.

Doctor: Let's take this step by step. What do you think you've ingested?

Patient: I'm not entirely sure, but there was an open cleaning product in the kitchen.

Doctor: I understand how worried you must be, and we're here to take care of you. Are you experiencing any nausea, vomiting, or dizziness?

Patient: Yes, and my stomach is in a lot of pain.

Doctor: We're going to act immediately to help you. We'll perform a gastric lavage and do some tests to find out what happened. Don't worry, you're in good hands, and we'll take good care of you.

Comprehension Questions

1. **What does the patient believe they have ingested?**
   a. Expired medication
   b. Spoiled food
   c. A toxic substance
   d. Excessive alcohol

2. **Where did the patient find the suspicious substance?**
   a. In the bathroom
   b. In the kitchen
   c. In the garden
   d. In the garage

3. **What medical procedure does the doctor mention?**
   a. A blood transfusion
   b. A gastric lavage
   c. An MRI
   d. An electrocardiogram

Answers

1. **c)** Una sustancia tóxica - A toxic substance
2. **b)** En la cocina - In the kitchen
3. **b)** Un lavado gástrico - A gastric lavage

Diálogo 8:
Dolor abdominal agudo - Acute Abdominal Pain

Paciente: Doctor, tengo un dolor fuerte y constante en mi abdomen.

Doctor: Lamento escuchar eso. Cuéntame más sobre ese dolor.

Paciente: Es un dolor agudo y no me da descanso. Lo siento mucho aquí, en la parte baja derecha de mi abdomen.

Doctor: Eso suena preocupante. ¿Has tenido fiebre o náuseas últimamente?

Paciente: Sí, y el dolor me dificulta comer con normalidad.

Doctor: Podría ser apendicitis. Vamos a realizar un ultrasonido y unos análisis de sangre para confirmar. Tranquilo, estamos aquí para ayudarte.

Preguntas de comprensión

1. **¿Cómo describe el paciente el dolor?**
   a. Dolor leve y esporádico
   b. Dolor agudo y constante
   c. Dolor ardoroso y generalizado
   d. Dolor sordo y localizado

2. **¿Dónde localiza el paciente el dolor?**
   a. Parte inferior derecha del abdomen
   b. Parte superior izquierda del abdomen
   c. Todo el abdomen
   d. Lado izquierdo del abdomen

3. **¿Qué sospecha el doctor que podría ser la causa?**
   a. Gastritis
   b. Cálculos renales
   c. Apendicitis
   d. Úlcera estomacal

Dialogue 8:
Acute Abdominal Pain - Dolor abdominal agudo

Patient: Doctor, I have a severe, ongoing pain in my abdomen.

Doctor: I'm sorry to hear that. Tell me more about the pain.

Patient: It's sharp and relentless. I feel it intensely right here, in the lower right side of my abdomen.

Doctor: That sounds concerning. Have you experienced any fever or nausea recently?

Patient: Yes, and the pain is affecting my eating.

Doctor: It could be appendicitis. We're going to do an ultrasound and some blood tests to confirm. Don't worry, we are here to help you.

Comprehension Questions

1. **How does the patient describe the pain?**
   a. Mild and sporadic pain
   b. Sharp and constant pain
   c. Burning and widespread pain
   d. Dull and localized pain

2. **Where does the patient experience the pain?**
   a. Lower right part of the abdomen
   b. Upper left part of the abdomen
   c. All over the abdomen
   d. Left side of the abdomen

3. **What does the doctor suspect might be the cause?**
   a. Gastritis
   b. Kidney stones
   c. Appendicitis
   d. Stomach ulcer

Answers

1. **b)** Dolor agudo y constante - Sharp and constant pain
2. **a)** Parte inferior derecha del abdomen - Lower right part of the abdomen
3. **c)** Apendicitis - Appendicitis

Chronic Care:
Long-term management, Patient Education, and Follow-ups

Chronic care requires not only medical expertise but also a continuity of communication. In this set of dialogues, you'll delve into the language of long-term care management, from diabetes to hypertension. You'll gain the phrases necessary to educate patients, discuss ongoing treatment plans, and conduct follow-up discussions. These conversations will help you build trusting relationships with patients managing chronic conditions.

Manejo de la diabetes - Diabetes Management

Paciente: Doctor, me está costando mucho controlar mi diabetes.

Doctor: Comprendo que puede ser desafiante. Cuéntame, ¿cómo has estado midiendo tus niveles de azúcar en sangre?

Paciente: Uso un glucómetro, pero hay veces que se me olvida.

Doctor: Recuerda que es crucial hacerlo con regularidad para mantener tu salud. Hablemos sobre tu dieta. ¿Cómo te has estado alimentando?

Paciente: Trato de comer saludable, pero a veces es difícil.

Doctor: Es normal enfrentar desafíos. Vamos a ver juntos cómo mejorar tu dieta y cómo la alimentación y el ejercicio pueden ser tus aliados en el manejo de la diabetes.

Preguntas de comprensión

1. **¿Qué problema tiene el paciente?**
   a. Dificultad para controlar su diabetes
   b. Problemas de visión
   c. Dolores de cabeza frecuentes
   d. Pérdida de peso inexplicable

2. **¿Qué usa el paciente para monitorear su diabetes?**
   a. Un termómetro
   b. Un glucómetro
   c. Una aplicación de salud
   d. Revisiones médicas regulares

3. **¿Sobre qué hablarán el doctor y el paciente?**
   a. Cambio de medicamento
   b. Cirugía
   c. Tratamientos alternativos
   d. Plan de alimentación y ejercicio

Diabetes Management - Manejo de la diabetes

Patient: Doctor, I'm finding it really hard to manage my diabetes.

Doctor: I understand it can be challenging. Tell me, how have you been measuring your blood sugar levels?

Patient: I use a glucometer, but sometimes I forget.

Doctor: Remember, it's crucial to do it regularly for your health. Let's talk about your diet. How have you been eating?

Patient: I try to eat healthily, but sometimes I face difficulties.

Doctor: It's normal to face challenges. Let's look together at how to improve your diet and how food and exercise can be your allies in managing diabetes.

Comprehension Questions

1. **What problem is the patient having?**
   a. Difficulty controlling their diabetes
   b. Vision problems
   c. Frequent headaches
   d. Unexplained weight loss

2. **What does the patient use to monitor their diabetes?**
   a. A thermometer
   b. A glucometer
   c. A health app
   d. Regular medical check-ups

3. **What will the doctor and patient discuss?**
   a. Changing medication
   b. Surgery
   c. Alternative treatments
   d. Eating plan and exercise

Answers

1. **a)** Dificultad para controlar su diabetes - Difficulty controlling their diabetes
2. **b)** Un glucómetro - A glucometer
3. **d)** Plan de alimentación y ejercicio - Eating plan and exercise

Diálogo 10: Seguimiento de la hipertensión - Hypertension Follow-Up

Paciente: Hola, doctor. Estoy aquí para mi revisión de la hipertensión.

Doctor: Hola, es un placer verte de nuevo. Vamos a ver cómo está tu presión arterial. ¿Has notado algún aumento recientemente?

Paciente: Sí, he estado revisándola en casa y a veces supera los 140/90.

Doctor: Ya veo. Es importante cuidar eso. ¿Has intentado hacer cambios en tu alimentación?

Paciente: He intentado reducir la sal, pero me está costando.

Doctor: Es un buen inicio reducir la sal. Posiblemente necesitemos ajustar tu medicamento. Además, dime, ¿has sentido dolores de cabeza o mareos últimamente?

Paciente: Ahora que lo mencionas, sí, he tenido algunos dolores de cabeza.

Preguntas de comprensión

1. **¿Para qué está el paciente en la consulta?**
   a. Control de diabetes
   b. Revisión de colesterol
   c. Seguimiento de la hipertensión
   d. Problemas de tiroides

2. **¿Qué ha observado el paciente sobre su presión arterial?**
   a. Es muy baja
   b. No la ha medido
   c. Está un poco alta
   d. Está normal

3. **¿Qué sugiere el doctor además de la dieta?**
   a. Realizar pruebas adicionales
   b. Cambiar completamente el estilo de vida
   c. Hacer más ejercicio
   d. Ajustar el medicamento

Hypertension Follow-Up - Seguimiento de la hipertensión

Patient: Hello, Doctor. I'm here for my hypertension check-up.

Doctor: Hello, it's good to see you again. Let's check your blood pressure. Have you noticed any increases lately?

Patient: Yes, I've been monitoring it at home and sometimes it goes over 140/90.

Doctor: I see. It's important we keep an eye on this. Have you tried changing your diet at all?

Patient: I've tried cutting down on salt, but it's been challenging.

Doctor: Cutting down on salt is a good start. We might need to adjust your medication. Also, have you experienced any headaches or dizziness recently?

Patient: Now that you mention it, yes, I've had a few headaches.

Comprehension Questions

1. **Why is the patient at the clinic?**
   a. Diabetes control
   b. Cholesterol check
   c. Hypertension follow-up
   d. Thyroid issues

2. **What has the patient noticed about their blood pressure?**
   a. It is very low
   b. They haven't measured it
   c. It is a bit high
   d. It is normal

3. **What does the doctor suggest in addition to diet?**
   a. Additional tests
   b. Completely changing lifestyle
   c. More exercise
   d. Adjusting medication

Answers

1. **c)** Hypertension follow-up - Seguimiento de la hipertensión
2. **c)** It is a bit high - Está un poco alta
3. **d)** Adjusting medication - Ajustar el medicamento

Control del asma - Asthma Maintenance

Paciente: Doctor, necesito ayuda para controlar mejor mi asma.

Doctor: ¿Qué tan frecuentemente necesita usar su inhalador de emergencia?

Paciente: Lo uso casi a diario. No puedo realizar mis actividades con normalidad por culpa del asma.

Doctor: Tener un plan de acción contra el asma es esencial. Vamos a revisar sus medicamentos preventivos y veremos cuáles pueden ser los desencadenantes de sus crisis.

Paciente: ¿Cree que hay alergenos que empeoran mi situación?

Doctor: Sí, es posible. También consideraremos hacer pruebas de alergia y veremos cómo podemos hacer cambios en su ambiente para ayudarle.

Preguntas de comprensión

1. **¿Qué problema tiene el paciente?**
   a. Dificultad para manejar el asma
   b. Infecciones respiratorias frecuentes
   c. Alergias severas
   d. Problemas cardíacos

2. **¿Qué indica el uso frecuente del inhalador?**
   a. El asma está bien controlada
   b. El asma no está bien controlada
   c. El inhalador no es efectivo
   d. El paciente es alérgico al inhalador

3. **¿Qué aspectos adicionales considerará el doctor?**
   a. Cambio de medicamento
   b. Pruebas de alergia y ajustes ambientales
   c. Cirugía
   d. Cambios en la dieta

Dialogue 11:
Asthma Maintenance - Control del asma

Patient: Doctor, I really need help to better manage my asthma.

Doctor: How often do you need to use your emergency inhaler?

Patient: I use it almost every day. Asthma prevents me from doing my daily activities normally.

Doctor: Having a well-defined asthma action plan is crucial. Let's review your preventive medications and discuss factors that might trigger your attacks.

Patient: Do you think allergens are making my condition worse?

Doctor: Yes, that's a possibility. We will also consider conducting allergy tests and seeing how we can adjust your environment to help.

Comprehension Questions

1. **What problem is the patient having?**
   a. Difficulty managing asthma
   b. Frequent respiratory infections
   c. Severe allergies
   d. Heart problems

2. **What does frequent use of the inhaler indicate?**
   a. Asthma is well-controlled
   b. Asthma is not well-controlled
   c. The inhaler is ineffective
   d. The patient is allergic to the inhaler

3. **What additional aspects will the doctor consider?**
   a. Changing medication
   b. Allergy testing and environmental adjustments
   c. Surgery
   d. Changes in diet

Answers

1. **a)** Dificultad para manejar el asma - Difficulty managing asthma
2. **b)** El asma no está bien controlada - Asthma is not well-controlled
3. **b)** Pruebas de alergia y ajustes ambientales - Allergy testing and environmental adjustments

Diálogo 12:

Manejo de la artritis - Arthritis Management

Paciente: Doctor, últimamente mi artritis me causa mucho dolor.

Doctor: Entiendo, debe ser difícil. ¿En qué áreas sientes más dolor?

Paciente: En mis manos y rodillas principalmente, y también están hinchadas.

Doctor: ¿Has estado tomando tus medicamentos antiinflamatorios regularmente?

Paciente: Sí, pero ya no me alivian como antes.

Doctor: Veamos qué podemos hacer. Puede ser necesario ajustar tu medicamento. También la fisioterapia podría ser muy beneficiosa. ¿Has probado ejercicios suaves o aplicar calor?

Paciente: No mucho, ¿realmente ayuda?

Doctor: Sí, esos métodos pueden ayudar a disminuir el dolor y mejorar tu movilidad. Además, mantener un peso saludable es esencial para tu bienestar.

Preguntas de comprensión

1. **¿Cuál es el principal problema del paciente?**
   a. Problemas de visión
   b. Pérdida de peso
   c. Dolor e hinchazón por artritis
   d. Dificultad para respirar

2. **¿Dónde siente más dolor el paciente?**
   a. En la espalda y cuello
   b. En las manos y rodillas
   c. En los pies y tobillos
   d. En los hombros y codos

3. **¿Qué recomienda el doctor además del medicamento?**
   a. Reposo absoluto
   b. Fisioterapia y ejercicios suaves
   c. Cambios en la dieta
   d. Más pruebas médicas

Arthritis Management - Manejo de la artritis

Patient: Doctor, my arthritis is causing me a lot of pain these days.

Doctor: I understand, it must be tough. Where are you experiencing the most pain?

Patient: Mostly in my hands and knees, and they're swollen.

Doctor: Have you been consistent with your anti-inflammatory medication?

Patient: Yes, but they don't seem to provide relief like they used to.

Doctor: Let's see what we can do. Adjusting your medication might be necessary. Physical therapy could also be very helpful. Have you tried gentle exercises or applying heat?

Patient: I haven't done that much; does it really help?

Doctor: Yes, those methods can help ease the pain and improve your mobility. Also, keeping a healthy weight is vital for your well-being.

Comprehension Questions

1. **What is the main problem of the patient?**
   a. Vision problems
   b. Weight loss
   c. Pain and swelling from arthritis
   d. Difficulty breathing

2. **Where does the patient feel the most pain?**
   a. In the back and neck
   b. In the hands and knees
   c. In the feet and ankles
   d. In the shoulders and elbows

3. **What does the doctor recommend in addition to medication?**
   a. Complete rest
   b. Physical therapy and gentle exercises
   c. Diet changes
   d. More medical tests

Answers

1. **c)** Dolor e hinchazón por artritis - Pain and swelling from arthritis
2. **b)** En las manos y rodillas - In the hands and knees
3. **b)** Fisioterapia y ejercicios suaves - Physical therapy and gentle exercises

Diálogo 13: Enfermedad renal crónica - Chronic Kidney Disease

Paciente: Doctor, tengo enfermedad renal crónica y estoy preocupado por su progresión.

Doctor: ¿Ha notado algún cambio en sus síntomas o en cómo se siente en general?

Paciente: Últimamente me siento más cansado y he notado hinchazón en las piernas.

Doctor: Eso podría indicar que la función renal está empeorando. ¿Cómo ha estado su presión arterial?

Paciente: Ha estado alta. También me ha costado dormir.

Doctor: Es fundamental controlar la presión arterial. Revisaremos y ajustaremos sus medicamentos. Seguir una dieta adecuada también es importante.

Paciente: ¿Debo cambiar mi dieta?

Doctor: Sí, una dieta baja en sal y proteínas ayudará a sus riñones.

Preguntas de comprensión

1. **¿Cuál es la condición del paciente?**
   a. Insuficiencia cardíaca
   b. Enfermedad renal crónica
   c. Hipertensión
   d. Diabetes

2. **¿Qué síntomas ha experimentado el paciente?**
   a. Pérdida de peso y náuseas
   b. Cansancio e hinchazón en las piernas
   c. Dolor de cabeza y visión borrosa
   d. Fiebre y tos

3. **¿Qué recomienda el doctor para manejar la enfermedad?**
   a. Cambios en la dieta y ajuste de medicamentos
   b. Ejercicio intenso
   c. Cirugía
   d. Terapia de oxígeno

Chronic Kidney Disease - Enfermedad renal crónica

Patient: Doctor, I have chronic kidney disease and I'm concerned about its progression.

Doctor: Have you noticed any changes in your symptoms or how you feel overall?

Patient: I've been feeling more tired lately and noticed swelling in my legs.

Doctor: Those symptoms could indicate worsening kidney function. How about your blood pressure?

Patient: It's been high, and I've been having trouble sleeping.

Doctor: Controlling blood pressure is key. We'll review and possibly adjust your medications. It's also important to follow a suitable diet.

Patient: Should I change my diet?

Doctor: Yes, a diet low in salt and protein will help your kidneys.

Comprehension Questions

1. **What is the patient's condition?**
   a. Heart failure
   b. Chronic kidney disease
   c. Hypertension
   d. Diabetes

2. **What symptoms has the patient experienced?**
   a. Weight loss and nausea
   b. Tiredness and swelling in the legs
   c. Headache and blurred vision
   d. Fever and cough

3. **What does the doctor recommend for managing the disease?**
   a. Diet changes and medication adjustment
   b. Intense exercise
   c. Surgery
   d. Oxygen therapy

Answers

1. **b)** Enfermedad renal crónica - Chronic kidney disease
2. **b)** Cansancio e hinchazón en las piernas - Tiredness and swelling in the legs
3. **a)** Cambios en la dieta y ajuste de medicamentos - Diet changes and medication adjustment

Seguimiento de enfermedad cardíaca - Heart Disease Follow-Up

Paciente: Buenos días, Doctor. Estoy aquí para mi control de enfermedad cardíaca.

Doctor: Buenos días. Cuénteme, ¿cómo se ha sentido desde la última vez?

Paciente: He tenido episodios de dolor en el pecho y me canso con facilidad.

Doctor: ¿Ha seguido las indicaciones sobre dieta y ejercicio?

Paciente: Lo he intentado, pero me cuesta mantener la dieta.

Doctor: Es vital para su corazón. ¿Cómo han estado su presión arterial y su colesterol?

Paciente: La presión arterial está mejor, pero no he revisado el colesterol.

Doctor: Hagamos un análisis de sangre para ver el colesterol y revisemos sus medicamentos. Evitar el estrés y el tabaco también son clave.

Preguntas de comprensión

1. **¿Por qué acude el paciente al doctor?**
   a. Seguimiento de enfermedad cardíaca
   b. Control de peso
   c. Revisión de diabetes
   d. Problemas respiratorios

2. **¿Qué síntomas ha experimentado el paciente?**
   a. Problemas de visión
   b. Insomnio y ansiedad
   c. Dolores de cabeza y mareos
   d. Dolor en el pecho y fatiga

3. **¿Qué aspectos adicionales evaluará el doctor?**
   a. Pruebas de función pulmonar
   b. Examen de la vista
   c. Presión arterial y análisis de colesterol
   d. Actividad física y nivel de estrés

Dialogue 14:
Heart Disease Follow-Up - Seguimiento de enfermedad cardíaca

Patient: Good morning, Doctor. I'm here for my heart disease check-up.

Doctor: Good morning. Tell me, how have you been since our last meeting?

Patient: I've had some chest pain episodes and get easily tired.

Doctor: Have you been following the diet and exercise recommendations?

Patient: I've tried, but sticking to the diet is hard.

Doctor: It's crucial for your heart health. How about your blood pressure and cholesterol?

Patient: My blood pressure has gotten better, but I haven't checked my cholesterol.

Doctor: Let's do a blood test for cholesterol and review your medication. Also, remember that avoiding stress and smoking is important.

Comprehension Questions

1. **Why is the patient visiting the doctor?**
   a. Heart disease follow-up
   b. Weight control
   c. Diabetes check-up
   d. Respiratory problems

2. **What symptoms has the patient experienced?**
   a. Vision problems
   b. Insomnia and anxiety
   c. Headaches and dizziness
   d. Chest pain and fatigue

3. **What additional aspects will the doctor evaluate?**
   a. Lung function tests
   b. Eye examination
   c. Blood pressure and cholesterol test
   d. Physical activity and stress level

Answers

1. **a)** Seguimiento de enfermedad cardíaca - Heart disease follow-up
2. **d)** Dolor en el pecho y fatiga - Chest pain and fatigue
3. **c)** Presión arterial y análisis de colesterol - Blood pressure and cholesterol test

Pediatric Care:
Health Concerns in Children, Vaccinations, Parental Guidance

Caring for children presents unique challenges and requires a gentle, reassuring approach. This collection of dialogues provides you with the Spanish terminology and expressions needed to address pediatric concerns, discuss vaccinations, and offer guidance to parents. Learn how to navigate conversations about common childhood illnesses, ear infections, and asthma, ensuring you can support both young patients and their families with care and competence.

Diálogo 15:
Vacunación infantil - Childhood Vaccination

Madre: Buenos días, doctor. Estamos aquí para vacunar a nuestro hijo.

Doctor: Buenos días. ¿Cuántos años tiene su hijo?

Padre: Cuatro años.

Doctor: Perfecto, es la edad adecuada para varias vacunas importantes. ¿Ha tenido reacciones a vacunas anteriores?

Madre: No, todo ha ido bien.

Doctor: Excelente. Hoy le pondremos las vacunas contra sarampión, paperas, rubéola y varicela.

Padre: ¿Estas vacunas son seguras?

Doctor: Sí, son seguras y muy eficaces para prevenir estas enfermedades. Es crucial seguir el calendario de vacunación.

Preguntas de comprensión

1. **¿Por qué están en la consulta el padre, la madre y el niño?**
   a. Control de crecimiento
   b. Vacunación infantil
   c. Alergias
   d. Problemas de salud general

2. **¿Qué vacunas se aplicarán hoy?**
   a. Tétanos y difteria
   b. Hepatitis y gripe
   c. Polio y rotavirus
   d. Sarampión, paperas, rubéola y varicela

3. **¿Qué opina el doctor sobre la seguridad de las vacunas?**
   a. No son necesarias
   b. Son riesgosas pero necesarias
   c. Son seguras y efectivas
   d. No hay suficiente información

Childhood Vaccination - Vacunación infantil

Mother: Good morning, Doctor. We're here for our child's vaccinations.

Doctor: Good morning. How old is your child?

Father: He's four years old.

Doctor: Perfect, that's the right age for several key vaccinations. Has he had any reactions to previous vaccines?

Mother: No, everything has been fine so far.

Doctor: Great. Today, we'll administer the measles, mumps, rubella, and chickenpox vaccines.

Father: Are these vaccines safe?

Doctor: Yes, they're very safe and effective in preventing these diseases. Keeping up to date with the vaccination schedule is important.

Comprehension Questions

1. **Why are the father, mother, and child at the clinic?**
   a. Growth check-up
   b. Childhood vaccination
   c. Allergies
   d. General health issues

2. **What vaccines will be administered today?**
   a. Tetanus and diphtheria
   b. Hepatitis and flu
   c. Polio and rotavirus
   d. Measles, mumps, rubella, and chickenpox

3. **What is the doctor's opinion on the safety of the vaccines?**
   a. Not necessary
   b. Risky but necessary
   c. Safe and effective
   d. Not enough information

Answers

1. **b)** Vacunación infantil - Childhood vaccination
2. **d)** Sarampión, paperas, rubéola y varicela - Measles, mumps, rubella, and chickenpox
3. **c)** Son seguras y efectivas - Safe and effective

Diálogo 16:
Resfriado común infantil - Common Cold in Children

Madre: Doctor, creo que mi hijo tiene un resfriado. Está tosiendo y estornudando bastante.

Doctor: ¿Desde cuándo tiene estos síntomas?

Madre: Comenzaron hace unos tres días.

Doctor: ¿Ha tenido fiebre o problemas para respirar?

Padre: No ha tenido fiebre, pero le cuesta respirar por la nariz.

Doctor: Parece un resfriado común. Asegúrese de que descanse y beba suficientes líquidos. ¿Ha estado cerca de otros niños enfermos?

Madre: Sí, en su colegio hay varios niños resfriados.

Doctor: Es típico en las escuelas. Manténgalo en casa hasta que se recupere y recuerden lavarse las manos para evitar contagios.

Preguntas de comprensión

1. **¿Qué síntomas tiene el niño?**
   a. Fiebre alta y escalofríos
   b. Tos y estornudos
   c. Dolor de estómago y vómitos
   d. Erupción cutánea y picazón

2. **¿Cuánto tiempo hace que el niño tiene síntomas?**
   a. Una semana
   b. Un día
   c. Tres días
   d. Dos semanas

3. **¿Qué recomendaciones da el doctor para el cuidado del niño?**
   a. Cambios en la dieta
   b. Descanso, líquidos y permanecer en casa
   c. Antibióticos y reposo en cama
   d. Vacunas adicionales

Common Cold in Children - Resfriado común infantil

Mother: Doctor, I think my son has a cold. He's coughing and sneezing a lot.

Doctor: How long has he had these symptoms?

Mother: They started about three days ago.

Doctor: Has he had any fever or trouble breathing?

Father: No fever, but he's having trouble breathing through his nose.

Doctor: Sounds like a common cold. Ensure he gets plenty of rest and fluids. Has he been around other sick children recently?

Mother: Yes, several kids at his school have colds.

Doctor: That's common in school settings. Keep him home until he recovers and remember to wash hands frequently to prevent spread.

Comprehension Questions

1. **What symptoms does the child have?**
   a. High fever and chills
   b. Coughing and sneezing
   c. Stomach pain and vomiting
   d. Skin rash and itching

2. **How long has the child been showing symptoms?**
   a. One week
   b. One day
   c. Three days
   d. Two weeks

3. **What recommendations does the doctor give for the child's care?**
   a. Diet changes
   b. Rest, fluids, and staying at home
   c. Antibiotics and bed rest
   d. Additional vaccinations

Answers

1. **b)** Tos y estornudos - Coughing and sneezing
2. **c)** Tres días - Three days
3. **b)** Descanso, líquidos y permanecer en casa - Rest, fluids, and staying at home

Diálogo 17:
Infección ótica - Ear Infection

Padre: Doctor, mi hija tiene dolor en el oído y estoy preocupado.

Doctor: Entiendo tu preocupación. ¿Cuándo empezó a sentir dolor?

Padre: Hace dos días y parece que está empeorando.

Doctor: Vamos a ver. ¿Ha tenido fiebre o alguna secreción en el oído?

Madre: Sí, tuvo fiebre anoche y ha habido algo de líquido.

Doctor: Examinaremos sus oídos con cuidado. Parece una infección. ¿Ha tenido esto antes?

Madre: Ha tenido varias este año.

Doctor: Entonces debemos ser cuidadosos. Le recetaré un antibiótico y gotas. Es vital mantener el oído seco y limpio.

Preguntas de comprensión

1. **¿Qué síntoma presenta la niña?**
   a. Dolor de cabeza
   b. Dolor de oído
   c. Dolor de estómago
   d. Dolor de garganta

2. **¿Qué otros síntomas ha tenido la niña aparte del dolor?**
   a. Tos
   b. Sarpullido
   c. Fiebre y secreción en el oído
   d. Dolor en las articulaciones

3. **¿Qué tratamiento recetará el doctor?**
   a. Un antihistamínico
   b. Analgésicos
   c. Un antibiótico y gotas para el oído
   d. Medicamentos para la tos

Dialogue 17:
Ear Infection - Infección de oído

Father: Doctor, my daughter has pain in her ear, and I'm worried.

Doctor: I understand your concern. When did the pain start?

Father: About two days ago, and it seems to be getting worse.

Doctor: Let's take a look. Has she had a fever or any discharge from her ear?

Mother: Yes, she had a fever last night, and there's been some fluid.

Doctor: We'll carefully examine her ears. It looks like an infection. Has she had this before?

Mother: She's had a few this year.

Doctor: Then we need to treat it carefully. I'll prescribe an antibiotic and ear drops. Keeping her ear dry and clean is crucial.

Comprehension Questions

1. **What symptom is the girl experiencing?**
    - a. Headache
    - b. Ear pain
    - c. Stomach pain
    - d. Sore throat

2. **What other symptoms has the girl had besides pain?**
    - a. Cough
    - b. Rash
    - c. Fever and ear discharge
    - d. Joint pain

3. **What treatment will the doctor prescribe?**
    - a. An antihistamine
    - b. Painkillers
    - c. An antibiotic and ear drops
    - d. Cough medicine

Answers

1. **b)** Dolor de oído - Ear pain
2. **c)** Fiebre y secreción en el oído - Fever and ear discharge
3. **c)** Un antibiótico y gotas para el oído - An antibiotic and ear drops

Asma infantil - Childhood Asthma

Madre: Doctor, estoy preocupada por el asma de mi hijo. Ha tenido más crisis últimamente.

Doctor: ¿Puede describir las crisis?

Madre: Se queda sin aire fácilmente y empieza a toser mucho.

Doctor: ¿Está usando un inhalador de rescate? ¿Con qué frecuencia?

Padre: Sí, lo usa casi todos los días ahora.

Doctor: Eso es demasiado frecuente. Necesitamos revisar su plan de manejo del asma. ¿Ha habido algún cambio en su entorno que pueda estar desencadenando los ataques?

Madre: Recientemente empezó a jugar fútbol, y parece que después de jugar es cuando tiene más problemas.

Doctor: El ejercicio puede desencadenar asma en algunos niños. Vamos a ajustar su medicamento y considerar un plan de acción para cuando haga ejercicio.

Preguntas de comprensión

1. **¿Cuál es la preocupación de la madre?**
   a. Problemas de sueño
   b. Alergias
   c. Aumento en las crisisde asma
   d. Dolores de crecimiento

2. **¿Qué desencadena aparentemente las crisisde asma del niño?**
   a. Alimentos específicos
   b. Jugar al fútbol
   c. Animales domésticos
   d. El clima frío

3. **¿Qué plan propone el doctor?**
   a. Evitar el ejercicio
   b. Cambiar de escuela
   c. Ajustar el medicamentoy hacer un plan para el ejercicio
   d. Realizar pruebas de alergia

Childhood Asthma - Asma infantil

Mother: Doctor, I'm concerned about my son's asthma. He's been having more attacks lately.

Doctor: Can you describe these attacks?

Mother: He gets out of breath easily and starts coughing a lot.

Doctor: Is he using a rescue inhaler? How often?

Father: Yes, he's using it almost every day now.

Doctor: That's quite frequent. We need to review his asthma management plan. Has there been any change in his environment that might be triggering the attacks?

Mother: He recently started playing soccer, and it seems like after playing is when he has more problems.

Doctor: Exercise can trigger asthma in some children. We'll adjust his medication and consider an action plan for when he exercises.

Comprehension Questions

1. **What is the mother's concern?**
   a. Sleep problems
   b. Allergies
   c. Increase in asthma attacks
   d. Growing pains

2. **What apparently triggers the child's asthma attacks?**
   a. Specific foods
   b. Playing soccer
   c. Household pets
   d. Cold weather

3. **What plan does the doctor propose?**
   a. Avoid exercise
   b. Change schools
   c. Adjust medication and a plan for exercise
   d. Conduct allergy tests

Answers

1. **c)** Aumento en las crisis de asma - Increase in asthma attacks
2. **b)** Jugar al fútbol - Playing soccer
3. **c)** Ajustar el medicamentoy crear un plan para el ejercicio - Adjust medication and a plan for exercise

Consejos de nutrición infantil - Nutritional Advice for Children

Padre: Doctor, quiero que mis hijos coman de manera saludable. ¿Puede darnos algunos consejos?

Doctor: Por supuesto, una buena nutrición es esencial para su crecimiento. ¿Qué comen normalmente?

Madre: Cereal para el desayuno, un sándwich para el almuerzo y pollo con verduras para la cena.

Doctor: Es un buen comienzo. Asegúrense de incluir frutas y verduras variadas. ¿Comen algo entre comidas?

Padre: Suelen comer galletas o papas fritas.

Doctor: Prueben con bocadillos más saludables como yogur, frutas o nueces. ¿Y qué beben?

Madre: Principalmente jugos y a veces refrescos.

Doctor: Sería mejor reducir los jugos y refrescos y aumentar el consumo de agua.

Preguntas de comprensión

1. **¿Cuál es la preocupación del padre?**
   a. La cantidad de comida que comen los niños
   b. La calidad nutricional de la comida
   c. Alergias alimentarias
   d. El precio de los alimentos

2. **¿Qué tipo de bocadillos suelen comer los niños?**
   a. Galletas y papas fritas
   b. Frutas y verduras
   c. Yogur y nueces
   d. Pan y queso

3. **¿Qué cambio en la bebida recomienda el doctor?**
   a. Más jugos naturales
   b. Limitar jugos y refrescos
   c. Solo leche
   d. Bebidas energéticas

Nutritional Advice for Children - Consejos de nutrición infantil

Father: Doctor, I want to ensure my children are eating healthily. Can you give us some advice?

Doctor: Of course, good nutrition is crucial for their growth. What do they usually eat?

Mother: They have cereal for breakfast, a sandwich for lunch, and chicken with vegetables for dinner.

Doctor: That's a good start. Make sure to include a variety of fruits and vegetables. Do they snack between meals?

Father: They often eat cookies or chips.

Doctor: Try healthier snack options like yogurt, fruits, or nuts. And what about their drinks?

Mother: They mainly drink juices and sometimes sodas.

Doctor: It's better to reduce juices and sodas and encourage water intake.

Comprehension Questions

1. **What is the father's concern?**
   a. The amount of food the children eat
   b. The nutritional quality of the food
   c. Food allergies
   d. The cost of food

2. **What type of snacks do the children usually eat?**
   a. Cookies and chips
   b. Fruits and vegetables
   c. Yogurt and nuts
   d. Bread and cheese

3. **What change in drinks does the doctor recommend?**
   a. More natural juices
   b. Limit juices and sodas
   c. Only milk
   d. Energy drinks

Answers

1. **b)** La calidad nutricional de la comida - The nutritional quality of the food
2. **a)** Galletas y papas fritas - Cookies and chips
3. **b)** Limitar jugos y refrescos - Limit juices and sodas

Women's Health:
Prenatal Care, Gynecological Visits, and Family Planning

Women's health encompasses a range of vital topics that require sensitive and informed communication. Through these dialogues, you'll explore the language of prenatal check-ups, postpartum care, and family planning. Enhance your ability to provide compassionate guidance on contraception, discuss menopause symptoms, and lead routine gynecological exams. These scenarios are designed to give you the confidence to support women's health needs with clarity and empathy.

Control prenatal - Prenatal Check-Up

Paciente: Hola, doctora. Vengo por mi control prenatal.

Doctora: Hola. ¿Cómo te has sentido durante tu embarazo?

Paciente: Bien, aunque a veces tengo náuseas matutinas.

Doctora: Es común en el embarazo. ¿Estás tomando vitaminas prenatales?

Paciente: Sí, todos los días.

Doctora: Perfecto. Hoy revisaremos tu presión arterial y haremos un ultrasonidopara ver cómo está el bebé.

Paciente: ¿Con qué frecuencia debo tener controles prenatales?

Doctora: En general, son mensuales al principio del embarazo, y conforme éste avanza, se hacen con mayor frecuencia.

Preguntas de comprensión

1. **¿Por qué visita la paciente a la doctora?**
   - a. Dolor de espalda
   - b. Consejos de alimentación
   - c. Control prenatal
   - d. Náuseas matutinas

2. **¿Qué está tomando la paciente durante el embarazo?**
   - a. Antidepresivos
   - b. Suplementos de hierro
   - c. Medicamentos para el dolor
   - d. Vitaminas prenatales

3. **¿Qué hará la doctora durante la visita?**
   - a. Aplicar una vacuna
   - b. Recetar medicamentos
   - c. Programar una cirugía
   - d. Revisar la presión arterial y hacer un ultrasonido

Prenatal Check-Up - Control prenatal

Patient: Hello, Doctor. I'm here for my prenatal check-up.

Doctor: Hello. How have you been feeling during your pregnancy?

Patient: Good, though I sometimes have morning sickness.

Doctor: That's typical in pregnancy. Are you taking prenatal vitamins?

Patient: Yes, every day.

Doctor: Great. Today we'll check your blood pressure and perform an ultrasound to see how the baby is doing.

Patient: How often should I have prenatal check-ups?

Doctor: Generally, once a month at the beginning and more frequently as the pregnancy progresses.

Comprehension Questions

1. **Why is the patient visiting the doctor?**
   a. Back pain
   b. Dietary advice
   c. Prenatal check-up
   d. Morning sickness

2. **What is the patient taking during her pregnancy?**
   a. Antidepressants
   b. Iron supplements
   c. Painkillers
   d. Prenatal vitamins

3. **What will the doctor do during the visit?**
   a. Give a vaccine
   b. Prescribe medication
   c. Schedule surgery
   d. Check blood pressure and perform an ultrasound

Answers

1. **c)** Control prenatal - Prenatal check-up
2. **d)** Vitaminas prenatales - Prenatal vitamins
3. **d)** Revisar la presión arterial y hacer un ultrasonido- Check blood pressure and perform an ultrasound

Diálogo 21:
Cuidado posparto - Postpartum Care

Paciente: Hola, doctora. Vengo para mi revisión posparto.

Doctora: Hola. ¿Cómo te has sentido desde el parto?

Paciente: Estoy algo cansada y a veces siento dolor.

Doctora: Es normal después del parto. ¿Cómo va la lactancia?

Paciente: Va bien, aunque a veces duele.

Doctora: Es común al principio. Es importante alimentarse bien y descansar. ¿Has sentido tristeza o tenido cambios de humor?

Paciente: Sí, hay días que me siento triste.

Doctora: Es importante hablar de esos sentimientos. El apoyo emocional es clave en el cuidado posparto.

Preguntas de comprensión

1. **¿Cuál es el motivo de la visita de la paciente?**
   a. Dolor abdominal
   b. Revisión posparto
   c. Problemas de lactancia
   d. Control del embarazo

2. **¿Qué tema menciona la paciente sobre la lactancia?**
   a. Es dolorosa a veces
   b. No está lactando
   c. Es fácil
   d. Tiene mucha leche

3. **¿Qué aspecto emocional aborda la doctora?**
   a. Cambios de humor y tristeza
   b. Estrés
   c. Ansiedad
   d. Felicidad

Dialogue 21:
Postpartum Care - Cuidado posparto

Patient: Hello, Doctor. I've come for my postpartum check-up.

Doctor: Hello. How have you been feeling since giving birth?

Patient: I'm a bit tired and sometimes in pain.

Doctor: It's normal to feel this way after childbirth. How is breastfeeding going?

Patient: Well, but sometimes it's painful.

Doctor: That can happen at the beginning. It's important to eat well and get enough rest. Have you been experiencing mood swings or sadness?

Patient: Yes, some days I feel sad.

Doctor: It's important to talk about these feelings. Emotional support is a part of postpartum care.

Comprehension Questions

1. **Why is the patient visiting the doctor?**
   a. Abdominal pain
   b. Postpartum review
   c. Breastfeeding problems
   d. Pregnancy check-up

2. **What does the patient mention about breastfeeding?**
   a. It's painful sometimes
   b. She's not breastfeeding
   c. It's easy
   d. She has a lot of milk

3. **What emotional aspect does the doctor address?**
   a. Mood swings and sadness
   b. Stress
   c. Anxiety
   d. Happiness

Answers

1. **b)** Revisión posparto - Postpartum review
2. **a)** Es dolorosa a veces - It's painful sometimes
3. **a)** Cambios de humor y tristeza - Mood swings and sadness

Diálogo 22: Consulta sobre anticonceptivos - Contraception Consultation

Paciente: Hola, doctora. Quisiera información sobre métodos anticonceptivos.

Doctora: Por supuesto. ¿Tienes alguna preferencia o necesidad específica?

Paciente: No estoy segura. ¿Cuáles son las opciones?

Doctora: Hay varias opciones: píldoras, inyecciones, implantes, DIU y métodos de barrera, como los condones.

Paciente: ¿Cuál es el más efectivo?

Doctora: Los implantes y el DIU son muy efectivos, pero todo depende de tu estilo de vida y comodidad.

Paciente: ¿Y tienen efectos secundarios?

Doctora: Pueden variar. Las píldoras e inyecciones pueden afectar tu ciclo menstrual, por ejemplo. Es importante elegir el método que mejor se adapte a tus necesidades.

Preguntas de comprensión

1. **¿Acerca de qué desea saber la paciente?**
   a. Información sobre anticonceptivos
   b. Consejos de nutrición
   c. Tratamiento para infecciones
   d. Ejercicios para embarazadas

2. **¿Qué métodos anticonceptivos menciona la doctora?**
   a. Sólo píldoras
   b. Métodos naturales
   c. Píldoras, inyecciones, implantes, DIU, condones
   d. Sólo cirugía

3. **¿Qué considera la doctora importante al elegir un método anticonceptivo?**
   a. La efectividad y adaptación al estilo de vida
   b. La opinión de la pareja
   c. El costo
   d. La edad de la paciente

Contraception Consultation - Consulta sobre anticonceptivos

Patient: Hello, Doctor. I would like information about contraceptive methods.

Doctor: Of course. Do you have any specific preferences or needs?

Patient: I'm not sure. What are the options?

Doctor: There are several: pills, injections, implants, IUDs, and barrier methods like condoms.

Patient: Which is the most effective?

Doctor: Implants and IUDs are very effective, but it all depends on your lifestyle and comfort.

Patient: What about side effects?

Doctor: They can vary. Pills and injections can affect your menstrual cycle, for example. It's important to choose the method that best suits you.

Comprehension Questions

1. **What does the patient want to know?**
   a. Information about contraceptives
   b. Nutrition advice
   c. Treatment for infections
   d. Exercises for pregnancy

2. **What contraceptive methods does the doctor mention?**
   a. Only pills
   b. Natural methods
   c. Pills, injections, implants, IUDs, condoms
   d. Only surgery

3. **What does the doctor consider important when choosing a contraceptive method?**
   a. Effectiveness and adaptation to lifestyle
   b. Partner's opinion
   c. The cost
   d. The patient's age

Answers

1. **a)** Información sobre anticonceptivos - Information about contraceptives
2. **c)** Píldoras, inyecciones, implantes, DIU, condones - Pills, injections, implants, IUDs, condoms
3. **a)** La efectividad y adaptación al estilo de vida - Effectiveness and adaptation to lifestyle

Síntomas de la menopausia - Menopause Symptoms

Paciente: Doctora, creo que podría estar empezando la menopausia.

Doctora: ¿Qué síntomas estás teniendo?

Paciente: Tengo sofocos y cambios de humor. También mi periodo es irregular.

Doctora: Son síntomas comunes de la menopausia. ¿Has tenido problemas para dormir?

Paciente: Sí, y a veces me siento muy cansada durante el día.

Doctora: Eso también es típico. Podemos hablar sobre opciones para manejar los síntomas, como cambios en el estilo de vida y, si es necesario, tratamiento hormonal.

Paciente: ¿Hay algo más que deba hacer?

Doctora: Es importante mantener una dieta saludable, hacer ejercicio regularmente y cuidar tu salud mental.

Preguntas de comprensión

1. **¿Cuáles son los síntomas que la paciente cree que están relacionados con la menopausia?**
   a. Sofocos y cambios de humor
   b. Pérdida de cabello y uñas quebradizas
   c. Aumento de peso y visión borrosa
   d. Dolor de cabeza y fiebre

2. **¿Qué sugiere la doctora para manejar los síntomas?**
   a. Ignorarlos, ya que son normales
   b. Tomar más vitaminas
   c. Cambios en el estilo de vida y tratamiento hormonal
   d. Iniciar una dieta estricta

3. **¿Qué consejo adicional da la doctora?**
   a. Mantener una dieta saludable y ejercicio regular
   b. Reducir el consumo de agua
   c. Cambiar de trabajo
   d. Evitar salir con amigos

Menopause Symptoms - Síntomas de la menopausia

Patient: Doctor, I think I might be starting menopause.

Doctor: What symptoms are you experiencing?

Patient: I have hot flashes and mood swings. Also, my cycle is irregular.

Doctor: Those are common symptoms of menopause. Have you had trouble sleeping?

Patient: Yes, and sometimes I feel very tired during the day.

Doctor: That's also typical. We can discuss options for managing the symptoms, like lifestyle changes and, if necessary, hormonal treatment.

Patient: Is there anything else I should do?

Doctor: It's important to maintain a healthy diet, exercise regularly, and take care of your mental health.

Comprehension Questions

1. **What symptoms does the patient believe are related to menopause?**
   a. Hot flashes and mood swings
   b. Hair loss and brittle nails
   c. Weight gain and blurred vision
   d. Headache and fever

2. **What does the doctor suggest for managing the symptoms?**
   a. Ignore them as they are normal
   b. Take more vitamins
   c. Lifestyle changes and hormonal treatment
   d. Start a strict diet

3. **What additional advice does the doctor give?**
   a. Maintain a healthy diet and regular exercise
   b. Reduce water consumption
   c. Change jobs
   d. Avoid going out with friends

Answers

1. **a)** Sofocos y cambios de humor - Hot flashes and mood swings
2. **c)** Cambios en el estilo de vida y tratamiento hormonal - Lifestyle changes and hormonal treatment
3. **a)** Mantener una dieta saludable y ejercicio regular - Maintain a healthy diet and regular exercise

Examen ginecológico de rutina - Routine Gynecological Exam

Doctora: Hola, estoy aquí para tu examen ginecológico de rutina. ¿Cómo te has sentido últimamente?

Paciente: Hola, doctora. Me he sentido bien, no he tenido ninguna molestia.

Doctora: ¿Cuándo fue tu último periodo menstrual?

Paciente: Hace unas tres semanas.

Doctora: ¿Has tenido problemas ginecológicos antes o tienes antecedentes familiares que deberíamos conocer?

Paciente: No, todo ha sido normal hasta ahora.

Doctora: Durante el examen, revisaré tu salud reproductiva y realizaré una prueba de Papanicolaou. ¿Has notado algún cambio en tus mamas?

Paciente: No, todo parece normal.

Doctora: Excelente. Después del examen, hablaremos sobre cualquier recomendación o prueba adicional si es necesario.

Preguntas de comprensión

1. **¿Cuál es el motivo de consulta de la paciente?**
   a. Consulta por embarazo
   b. Examen ginecológico de rutina
   c. Dolor crónico
   d. Problemas de salud recientes

2. **¿Qué revisará la doctora durante el examen?**
   a. Salud reproductiva y prueba de Papanicolaou
   b. Sólo la presión arterial
   c. Niveles de azúcar en la sangre
   d. Problemas de la piel

3. **¿Qué pregunta la doctora sobre los antecedentes familiares?**
   a. Historial de diabetes
   b. Enfermedades cardíacas
   c. Antecedentes de alergias
   d. Problemas ginecológicos o antecedentes familiares

Routine Gynecological Exam - Examen ginecológico de rutina

Doctor: Hello, I'm here for your routine gynecological exam. How have you been feeling lately?

Patient: Hello, Doctor. I've been feeling fine, no specific issues.

Doctor: When was your last menstrual period?

Patient: About three weeks ago.

Doctor: Do you have any history of gynecological issues or family history that we should be aware of?

Patient: No, everything has been normal so far.

Doctor: During the exam, I'll check your reproductive health and perform a Pap smear. Have you noticed any changes in your breasts?

Patient: No, everything seems normal.

Doctor: Excellent. After the exam, we'll discuss any recommendations or further tests if necessary.

Comprehension Questions

1. **What is the reason for the patient's visit?**
   a. Pregnancy consultation
   b. Routine gynecological exam
   c. Chronic pain
   d. Recent health problems

2. **What will the doctor check during the exam?**
   a. Reproductive health and Pap smear
   b. Only blood pressure
   c. Blood sugar levels
   d. Skin problems

3. **What does the doctor ask about family history?**
   a. History of diabetes
   b. Heart diseases
   c. Allergy history
   d. Gynecological problems or family history

Answers

1. **b)** Examen ginecológico de rutina - Routine gynecological exam
2. **a)** Salud reproductiva y prueba de Papanicolaou - Reproductive health and Pap smear
3. **d)** Problemas ginecológicos o antecedentes familiares - Gynecological problems or family history

Geriatric Care:
Elderly Patient Care, Management of Age-Related Conditions

Geriatric care is a practice of patience, understanding, and comprehensive communication. These dialogues immerse you in the nuances of caring for the elderly, addressing common age-related conditions such as Alzheimer's, arthritis, and vision and hearing loss. You will acquire the language skills to manage these sensitive conversations, ensuring you provide the reassurance and clear instructions that enhance the quality of life for older adults.

Seguimiento del alzheimer - Alzheimer's Follow-Up

Doctor: Buenos días, estamos aquí para su seguimiento del Alzheimer. ¿Cómo se ha sentido?

Paciente: Buenos días. Últimamente me cuesta recordar cosas.

Doctor: ¿Ha tenido cambios en su rutina diaria o en su estado de ánimo?

Paciente: Sí, a veces me siento confundido y me irrito con facilidad.

Doctor: Es importante mantener una rutina regular. ¿Cómo va con sus medicamentos?

Paciente: A veces olvido tomarlos.

Doctor: Podemos considerar un organizador de medicamentos. ¿Está recibiendo apoyo de sus familiares?

Paciente: Sí, mi familia me ayuda mucho.

Doctor: Eso es bueno. También le recomendamos actividades que estimulen la mente, como rompecabezas o lectura.

Preguntas de comprensión

1. **¿Cuál es el motivo de consulta del paciente?**
   a. Seguimiento del Alzheimer
   b. Control de diabetes
   c. Dolor en las articulaciones
   d. Revisión de la presión arterial

2. **¿Qué problema menciona el paciente?**
   a. Dificultades para dormir
   b. Pérdida de audición
   c. Cambios en la visión
   d. Dificultades para recordar

3. **¿Qué recomienda el doctor para ayudar con los medicamentos?**
   a. Dejar de tomarlos
   b. Cambiar el medicamento
   c. Usar un organizador de medicamentos
   d. Tomarlos sólo cuando sea necesario

Alzheimer's Follow-Up - Seguimiento del alzheimer

Doctor: Good morning, we are here for your Alzheimer's follow-up. How have you been feeling?

Patient: Good morning. Lately, I've been having trouble remembering things.

Doctor: Have you noticed any changes in your daily routine or mood?

Patient: Yes, I sometimes feel confused and get irritated easily.

Doctor: It's important to maintain a regular routine. How are you doing with your medications?

Patient: I sometimes forget to take them.

Doctor: We can consider using a medication organizer. Are you receiving support from family members?

Patient: Yes, my family helps me a lot.

Doctor: That's good. We also recommend activities that stimulate the mind, like puzzles or reading.

Comprehension Questions

1. **What is the reason for the patient's visit?**
   a. Alzheimer's follow-up
   b. Diabetes check-up
   c. Joint pain
   d. Blood pressure review

2. **What problem does the patient mention?**
   a. Difficulties sleeping
   b. Hearing loss
   c. Vision changes
   d. Difficulties remembering

3. **What does the doctor recommend to help with the medications?**
   a. Stop taking them
   b. Change the medication
   c. Use a medication organizer
   d. Take them only when necessary

Answers

1. **a)** Seguimiento del Alzheimer - Alzheimer's follow-up
2. **d)** Dificultades para recordar - Difficulties remembering
3. **c)** Usar un organizador de medicamentos - Use a medication organizer

Artritis en personas mayores - Arthritis in the Elderly

Doctor: Hola, he notado en su historial que tiene artritis. ¿Cómo ha estado manejando el dolor?

Paciente: Hola, doctor. El dolor en mis manos y rodillas ha sido más intenso últimamente.

Doctor: ¿Está tomando algún medicamento para la artritis?

Paciente: Sí, pero no siempre es efectivo.

Doctor: Podemos considerar ajustar su medicamento. ¿Ha intentado fisioterapia o ejercicios suaves?

Paciente: No mucho, me preocupa que el ejercicio empeore el dolor.

Doctor: El movimiento suave puede ayudar a aliviar el dolor. También es importante mantener un peso saludable.

Paciente: ¿Algún otro consejo?

Doctor: Aplicar calor o frío en las áreas afectadas puede ser útil, y mantenerse activo dentro de sus límites es clave.

Preguntas de comprensión

1. **¿Cuál es la condición médica del paciente?**
   a. Hipertensión
   b. Artritis
   c. Diabetes
   d. Problemas de visión

2. **¿Qué problema tiene el paciente con su medicamento actual?**
   a. Es muy caro
   b. Causa somnolencia
   c. No siempre es efectivo
   d. Es muy efectivo

3. **¿Qué sugiere el doctor para manejar el dolor?**
   a. Ajustar el medicamento y realizar ejercicios suaves
   b. Dejar de moverse
   c. Cirugía
   d. Sólo descansar

Dialogue 26:
Arthritis in the Elderly - Artritis en personas mayores

Doctor: Hello, I see from your history that you have arthritis. How have you been managing the pain?

Patient: Hello, Doctor. The pain in my hands and knees has been more intense lately.

Doctor: Are you taking any medication for arthritis?

Patient: Yes, but it's not always effective.

Doctor: We can consider adjusting your medication. Have you tried physical therapy or gentle exercises?

Patient: Not much, I'm worried that exercise might make the pain worse.

Doctor: Gentle movement can actually help alleviate the pain. It's also important to maintain a healthy weight.

Patient: Any other advice?

Doctor: Applying heat or cold to the affected areas can be helpful. And staying active within your limits is key.

Comprehension Questions

1. **What is the patient's medical condition?**
   a. Hypertension
   b. Arthritis
   c. Diabetes
   d. Vision problems

2. **What issue does the patient have with their current medication?**
   a. It's very expensive
   b. It causes drowsiness
   c. It's not always effective
   d. It's very effective

3. **What does the doctor suggest for managing the pain?**
   a. Adjust the medication and gentle exercises
   b. Stop moving
   c. Surgery
   d. Just rest

Answers

1. **b)** Artritis - Arthritis
2. **c)** No siempre es efectivo - It's not always effective
3. **a)** Ajustar el medicamento y realizar ejercicios suaves - Adjust the medication and gentle exercises

Pérdida de audición en personas mayores - Hearing Loss in the Elderly

Doctor: Buenos días, veo que tiene problemas de audición. ¿Cuándo comenzó a notarlo?

Paciente: Buenos días, doctor. Empecé a tener dificultades hace unos meses.

Doctor: ¿Tiene problemas para escuchar en ambientes ruidosos o para llevar conversaciones?

Paciente: Sí, especialmente cuando hay mucho ruido de fondo.

Doctor: Podría ser útil realizar una prueba de audición. ¿Ha tenido exposición prolongada a ruidos fuertes?

Paciente: Trabajé en construcción, así que sí.

Doctor: La exposición a ruido puede afectar la audición. Vamos a programar una audiometría. Mientras tanto, usar un audífono podría ayudarle.

Paciente: ¿Hay algo más que pueda hacer?

Doctor: Es importante que evite ruidos fuertes y que proteja sus oídos. También, algunos ejercicios de rehabilitación auditiva pueden ser beneficiosos.

Preguntas de comprensión

1. **¿Cuál es la condición médica que se está evaluando?**
   a. Problemas de visión
   b. Artritis
   c. Pérdida de audición
   d. Diabetes

2. **¿Qué experiencia pasada del paciente podría haber contribuido al problema?**
   a. Exposición a ruidos fuertes
   b. Estrés
   c. Dieta pobre
   d. Falta de ejercicio

3. **¿Qué sugiere el doctor para ayudar con el problema?**
   a. Cambiar la dieta
   b. Tomar medicamentos
   c. Realizar más actividad física
   d. Usar un audífono y hacer ejercicios de rehabilitación auditiva

Dialogue 27:

Hearing Loss in the Elderly - Pérdida de audición en personas mayores

Doctor: Good morning, I've noticed that you have hearing problems. When did you start to notice it?

Patient: Good morning, Doctor. I started having difficulties a few months ago.

Doctor: Do you have trouble hearing in noisy environments or following conversations?

Patient: Yes, especially when there's a lot of background noise.

Doctor: It might be useful to have a hearing test. Have you had prolonged exposure to loud noises?

Patient: I worked in construction, so yes.

Doctor: Exposure to noise can affect hearing. Let's schedule an audiometry. Meanwhile, using a hearing aid might help.

Patient: Is there anything else I can do?

Doctor: Avoiding loud noises and protecting your ears is important. Also, some auditory rehabilitation exercises might be beneficial.

Comprehension Questions

1. **What medical condition is being evaluated?**
   a. Vision problems
   b. Arthritis
   c. Hearing loss
   d. Diabetes

2. **What past experience of the patient might have contributed to the issue?**
   a. Exposure to loud noises
   b. Stress
   c. Poor diet
   d. Lack of exercise

3. **What does the doctor suggest to help with the issue?**
   a. Change diet
   b. Take medication
   c. Do more physical activity
   d. Use a hearing aid and do auditory rehabilitation exercises

Answers

1. **c)** Pérdida de audición - Hearing loss
2. **a)** Exposición a ruidos fuertes - Exposure to loud noises
3. **d)** Usar un audífono y hacer ejercicios de rehabilitación auditiva - Use a hearing aid and do auditory rehabilitation exercises

Problemas de visión en personas mayores - Vision Problems in the Elderly

Doctor: Buenas tardes. ¿Cómo ha estado su visión recientemente?

Paciente: Buenas tardes, doctor. He notado que mi visión se está volviendo borrosa.

Doctor: ¿Tiene dificultades para leer o ver de lejos?

Paciente: Sí, sobre todo para leer letras pequeñas y durante la noche.

Doctor: Podría ser presbicia o cataratas. Vamos a hacerle un examen de la vista.

Paciente: ¿Necesitaré gafas?

Doctor: Es posible, dependerá de los resultados del examen. También es importante proteger sus ojos del sol y descansarlos regularmente.

Paciente: ¿Puede mejorar mi visión con el tiempo?

Doctor: El tratamiento adecuado puede ayudar a mantener su visión y prevenir el deterioro.

Preguntas de comprensión

1. **¿Qué problema está experimentando el paciente?**
   a. Visión borrosa
   b. Dolor en las articulaciones
   c. Pérdida de audición
   d. Problemas de memoria

2. **¿Qué condiciones sospecha el doctor?**
   a. Glaucoma y degeneración macular
   b. Presbicia y cataratas
   c. Diabetes e hipertensión
   d. Estrés y fatiga

3. **¿Qué recomendaciones da el doctor para el cuidado de los ojos?**
   a. Proteger los ojos del sol y descansarlos
   b. Usar gotas para los ojos constantemente
   c. Ejercicios oculares específicos
   d. Cambiar la dieta

Vision Problems in the Elderly - Problemas de visión en personas mayores

Doctor: Good afternoon. How has your vision been lately?

Patient: Good afternoon, Doctor. I've noticed that my vision is getting blurry.

Doctor: Do you have trouble reading or seeing things from a distance?

Patient: Yes, especially reading small print and at night.

Doctor: It could be presbyopia or cataracts. We'll do a vision exam.

Patient: Will I need glasses?

Doctor: It's possible, depending on the exam results. It's also important to protect your eyes from the sun and give them regular breaks.

Patient: Can my vision improve over time?

Doctor: Proper treatment can help maintain your vision and prevent further deterioration.

Comprehension Questions

1. **What problem is the patient experiencing?**
   a. Blurry vision
   b. Joint pain
   c. Hearing loss
   d. Memory problems

2. **What conditions does the doctor suspect?**
   a. Glaucoma and macular degeneration
   b. Presbyopia and cataracts
   c. Diabetes and hypertension
   d. Stress and fatigue

3. **What recommendations does the doctor give for eye care?**
   a. Protect eyes from the sun and give them rest
   b. Constantly use eye drops
   c. Specific eye exercises
   d. Change diet

Answers

1. **a)** Visión borrosa - Blurry vision
2. **b)** Presbicia y cataratas - Presbyopia and cataracts
3. **a)** Proteger los ojos del sol y descansarlos - Protect eyes from the sun and give them rest

Mental Health:
Discussing Mental Health Issues, Treatment, And Counseling

Discussing mental health requires a special blend of professionalism and empathy, particularly in a second language. These dialogues are crafted to guide you through the complexities of mental health conversations in Spanish, covering topics from anxiety and depression to stress management and sleep disorders. You'll learn how to approach sensitive subjects, offer support for treatment plans, and provide counseling with the appropriate terminology and tone to ensure understanding and compassion.

Consulta sobre la ansiedad - Anxiety Consultation

Doctor: Buenos días. Me comentaste que te sientes ansioso últimamente. Cuéntame más.

Paciente: Buenos días, Doctor. Sí, he estado sintiendo mucha ansiedad, especialmente en el trabajo.

Doctor: ¿Puedes describir los síntomas que experimentas?

Paciente: Tengo palpitaciones, sudoración y a veces me cuesta respirar.

Doctor: ¿Hay situaciones específicas que desencadenan tu ansiedad?

Paciente: Las reuniones y los plazos me hacen sentir muy nervioso.

Doctor: Es importante identificar las situaciones que provocan ansiedad para poder manejarlas mejor. ¿Has intentado alguna técnica de relajación?

Paciente: No realmente. No estoy seguro de qué hacer.

Doctor: Podemos hablar sobre técnicas de manejo del estrés y, si es necesario, explorar opciones de tratamiento como terapia o medicamentos.

Preguntas de comprensión

1. **¿Cuál es el motivo de consulta del paciente?**
   a. Problemas de sueño
   b. Ansiedad
   c. Problemas de audición
   d. Dolor crónico

2. **¿Qué síntomas menciona el paciente?**
   a. Pérdida de apetito
   b. Visión borrosa
   c. Palpitaciones y sudoración
   d. Dolores de cabeza

3. **¿Qué sugiere el doctor para manejar la ansiedad?**
   a. Técnicas de manejo del estrés y posiblemente terapia o medicamentos
   b. Cambiar de trabajo
   c. Ignorar los síntomas
   d. Hacer más ejercicio

Dialogue 29:
Anxiety Consultation - Consulta sobre la ansiedad

Doctor: Good morning. You mentioned that you have been feeling anxious lately. Tell me more.

Patient: Good morning, Doctor. Yes, I've been feeling a lot of anxiety, especially at work.

Doctor: Can you describe the symptoms you're experiencing?

Patient: I have heart palpitations, sweating, and sometimes I find it hard to breathe.

Doctor: Are there specific situations that trigger your anxiety?

Patient: Meetings and deadlines make me very nervous.

Doctor: It's important to identify situations that provoke anxiety so we can manage them better. Have you tried any relaxation techniques?

Patient: Not really. I'm not sure what to do.

Doctor: We can discuss stress management techniques and, if necessary, explore treatment options like therapy or medication.

Comprehension Questions

1. **What is the reason for the patient's visit?**
   a. Sleep problems
   b. Anxiety
   c. Hearing problems
   d. Chronic pain

2. **What symptoms does the patient mention?**
   a. Loss of appetite
   b. Blurry vision
   c. Heart palpitations and sweating
   d. Headaches

3. **What does the doctor suggest for managing anxiety?**
   a. Stress management techniques and possibly therapy or medication
   b. Change jobs
   c. Ignore the symptoms
   d. More exercise

Answers

1. **b)** Ansiedad - Anxiety
2. **c)** Palpitaciones y sudoración - Heart palpitations and sweating
3. **a)** Técnicas de manejo del estrés y posiblemente terapia o medicamentos - Stress management techniques and possibly therapy or medication

Seguimiento de la depresión - Depression Follow-Up

Doctor: ¿Cómo te has sentido desde la última consulta?

Paciente: Hola, doctor. Ha sido difícil. Aún me siento triste y desmotivado.

Doctor: ¿Aún tomas el medicamento que te receté?

Paciente: Sí, lo tomo todos los días, pero no veo mucha mejora.

Doctor: Quizás sea necesario ajustar o cambiar la dosis. ¿Cómo está tu sueño y apetito?

Paciente: Duermo mal y no tengo mucho apetito.

Doctor: Es importante que cuides tu sueño y nutrición. ¿Has intentado alguna actividad como ejercicio o pasatiempos?

Paciente: No realmente. No tengo energía para eso.

Doctor: Entiendo. Puede beneficiarte mucho el hacer ejercicio y realizar actividades que te gusten. Vamos a hablar también sobre la posibilidad de terapia.

Preguntas de comprensión

1. **¿Qué tipo de seguimiento tiene el paciente?**
   a. Control de artritis
   b. Seguimiento de la depresión
   c. Seguimiento de diabetes
   d. Revisión de hipertensión

2. **¿Qué problema tiene el paciente con el medicamento?**
   a. Es demasiado costoso
   b. No ve mucha mejora
   c. Le causa efectos secundarios
   d. Es difícil de encontrar

3. **¿Qué recomienda el doctor además del tratamiento médico?**
   a. Ejercicio y actividades que disfrute
   b. Solo seguir con el medicamento actual
   c. Cambiar completamente la dieta
   d. Viajar más

Depression Follow-Up - Seguimiento de la depresión

Doctor: How have you been feeling since our last meeting?

Patient: Hello, Doctor. It's been hard. I still feel sad and unmotivated.

Doctor: Are you continuing with the medication I prescribed?

Patient: Yes, I take it every day, but I don't see much improvement.

Doctor: Sometimes, adjusting the dosage or changing the medication can be necessary. How is your sleep and appetite?

Patient: I sleep poorly and don't have much of an appetite.

Doctor: It's important to take care of your sleep and nutrition. Have you tried any activities like exercise or hobbies?

Patient: Not really. I don't have the energy for that.

Doctor: I understand. Exercise and activities you enjoy can be very beneficial. We'll also talk about the possibility of therapy.

Comprehension Questions

1. **What kind of follow-up does the patient have?**
   a. Arthritis check
   b. Depression follow-up
   c. Diabetes follow-up
   d. Hypertension review

2. **What problem does the patient have with the medication?**
   a. Too expensive
   b. Doesn't see much improvement
   c. It causes side effects
   d. Hard to find

3. **What does the doctor recommend in addition to medical treatment?**
   a. Exercise and activities that are enjoyable
   b. Just continue with the current medication
   c. Completely change the diet
   d. Travel more

Answers

1. **b)** Seguimiento de la depresión - Depression follow-up
2. **b)** No ve mucha mejora - Doesn't see much improvement
3. **a)** Ejercicio y actividades que disfrute - Exercise and activities that are enjoyable

Diálogo 31:
Manejo del estrés - Stress Management

Doctor: Hola, veo en tus notas que has estado experimentando niveles altos de estrés. Háblame de ello.

Paciente: Hola, doctor. Sí, he estado bajo mucho estrés en el trabajo y en casa.

Doctor: ¿Qué síntomas de estrés has notado?

Paciente: Tengo dolores de cabeza frecuentes y me cuesta dormir.

Doctor: ¿Has probado alguna técnica de relajación o ejercicios para reducir el estrés?

Paciente: No mucho, no estoy seguro de qué hacer.

Doctor: La respiración profunda, la meditación y el ejercicio regular pueden ser útiles. ¿Cómo es tu rutina diaria?

Paciente: Bastante ocupada. No tengo mucho tiempo para mí.

Doctor: Es importante encontrar tiempo para relajarte y hacer actividades que disfrutes. Podemos hablar sobre gestionar tu tiempo y reducir el estrés.

Preguntas de comprensión

1. **¿Por qué visita el paciente al doctor?**
   a. Problemas de corazón
   b. Estrés
   c. Dolores de espalda
   d. Pérdida de audición

2. **¿Qué síntomas de estrés tiene el paciente?**
   a. Fiebre y escalofríos
   b. Dolores de cabeza y problemas para dormir
   c. Náuseas y mareos
   d. Pérdida de apetito

3. **¿Qué sugiere el doctor para reducir el estrés?**
   a. Tomar medicamentos
   b. Cambiar de trabajo
   c. Técnicas de relajación y gestión del tiempo
   d. Irse de vacaciones

Dialogue 31:
Stress Management - Manejo del estrés

Doctor: Hello, I see in your notes that you have been experiencing high levels of stress. Tell me about it.

Patient: Hello, Doctor. Yes, I've been under a lot of stress at work and at home.

Doctor: What stress symptoms have you noticed?

Patient: I frequently have headaches and find it hard to sleep.

Doctor: Have you tried any relaxation techniques or exercises to reduce stress?

Patient: Not much, I'm not sure what to do.

Doctor: Deep breathing, meditation, and regular exercise can be helpful. What is your daily routine like?

Patient: Quite busy. I don't have much time for myself.

Doctor: It's important to find time to relax and do activities you enjoy. We can discuss managing your time and reducing stress.

Comprehension Questions

1. **Why is the patient visiting the doctor?**
   a. Heart problems
   b. Stress
   c. Back pains
   d. Hearing loss

2. **What stress symptoms does the patient have?**
   a. Fever and chills
   b. Headaches and sleep problems
   c. Nausea and dizziness
   d. Loss of appetite

3. **What does the doctor suggest to reduce stress?**
   a. Take medication
   b. Change jobs
   c. Relaxation techniques and time management
   d. Go on vacation

Answers

1. **b)** Estrés - Stress
2. **b)** Dolores de cabeza y problemas para dormir - Headaches and sleep problems
3. **c)** Técnicas de relajación y gestión del tiempo - Relaxation techniques and time management

Trastornos del sueño - Sleep Disorders

Doctor: Buenas tardes. Me comentaste que tienes problemas para dormir. ¿Puedes darme más detalles?

Paciente: Buenas tardes, doctor. Sí, me cuesta mucho dormirme y me despierto varias veces durante la noche.

Doctor: ¿Desde cuándo tienes estos problemas de sueño?

Paciente: Ha empeorado en los últimos meses.

Doctor: ¿Tienes preocupaciones o estrés que puedan afectar tu sueño?

Paciente: Tengo mucho estrés en el trabajo. A veces pienso en eso cuando intento dormir.

Doctor: El estrés puede afectar seriamente el sueño. ¿Practicas alguna actividad relajante antes de acostarte?

Paciente: No realmente. Normalmente veo la televisión.

Doctor: Te recomendaría crear una rutina relajante antes de dormir. Evitar pantallas, leer un libro o escuchar música tranquila puede ayudar.

Preguntas de comprensión

1. **¿Cuál es el problema que tiene el paciente?**
   - a. Dolor de cabeza
   - b. Problemas de audición
   - c. Trastornos del sueño
   - d. Problemas de visión

2. **¿Qué afecta el sueño del paciente?**
   - a. Comer demasiado tarde
   - b. Estrés en el trabajo
   - c. Hacer mucho ejercicio
   - d. El clima

3. **¿Qué recomendación da el doctor para mejorar el sueño?**
   - a. Tomar medicamentos para dormir
   - b. Hacer una rutina relajante antes de dormir
   - c. Dormir más horas durante el día
   - d. Cambiar el colchón

Dialogue 32:
Sleep Disorders - Trastornos del sueño

Doctor: Good afternoon. You mentioned that you have trouble sleeping. Can you give me more details?

Patient: Good afternoon, Doctor. Yes, I have a hard time falling asleep and I wake up several times during the night.

Doctor: How long have you been having these sleep problems?

Patient: It's gotten worse in the last few months.

Doctor: Do you have worries or stress that might be affecting your sleep?

Patient: I have a lot of stress at work. Sometimes I think about that when I try to sleep.

Doctor: Stress can seriously affect sleep. Do you engage in any relaxing activities before bed?

Patient: Not really. I usually watch TV.

Doctor: I would recommend creating a relaxing routine before bed. Avoiding screens, reading a book, or listening to soft music can help.

Comprehension Questions

1. **What problem does the patient have?**
   a. Headache
   b. Hearing problems
   c. Sleep disorders
   d. Vision problems

2. **What affects the patient's sleep?**
   a. Eating too late
   b. Stress at work
   c. Doing a lot of exercise
   d. The weather

3. **What recommendation does the doctor give to improve sleep?**
   a. Take sleeping medication
   b. Have a relaxing routine before bed
   c. Sleep more hours during the day
   d. Change the mattress

Answers

1. **c)** Trastornos del sueño - Sleep disorders
2. **b)** Estrés en el trabajo - Stress at work
3. **b)** Hacer una rutina relajante antes de dormir - Have a relaxing routine before bed

Routine Check-Ups:
General Health Assessments and Vital Signs

Routine check-ups are a cornerstone of preventive medicine and patient care. In this segment, you will learn to discuss general health assessments and vital signs, the bread and butter of daily medical interactions. These dialogues will guide you through conducting an annual physical exam, checking blood pressure, and discussing cholesterol levels. Equipped with these conversational tools, you can ensure your patients stay informed about their health status and understand their test results.

Diálogo 33: Examen físico anual - Annual Physical Exam

Doctor: Buenos días. Hoy tenemos tu examen físico anual. ¿Cómo te has sentido este año?

Paciente: Buenos días, doctor. Me he sentido bastante bien, gracias.

Doctor: ¿Has tenido algún cambio significativo en tu salud o estilo de vida?

Paciente: No, todo ha sido bastante estable.

Doctor: Vamos a revisar tu peso, altura y presión arterial. También escucharé tu corazón y pulmones.

Paciente: ¿Necesitaré análisis de sangre?

Doctor: Sí, haremos análisis de sangre para revisar tu colesterol y niveles de azúcar.

Paciente: ¿Debo hacer algo en particular después del examen?

Doctor: Sólo mantener un estilo de vida saludable y seguir cualquier recomendación específica que surja del examen.

Preguntas de comprensión

1. **¿Cuál es el propósito de la visita?**
   a. Revisión de la vista
   b. Examen físico anual
   c. Consulta por dolor
   d. Revisión de la audición

2. **¿Qué revisará el doctor en el examen?**
   a. Sólo la presión arterial
   b. Niveles de estrés
   c. Peso, altura, presión arterial, corazón y pulmones
   d. Historial familiar

3. **¿Qué análisis adicionales ordenará el doctor?**
   a. Análisis de sangre para colesterol y glucosa
   b. Resonancia magnética
   c. Electrocardiograma
   d. Pruebas de alergia

Annual Physical Exam - Examen físico anual

Doctor: Good morning. Today we have your annual physical exam. How have you been feeling this year?

Patient: Good morning, Doctor. I've been feeling pretty good, thank you.

Doctor: Have you had any significant changes in your health or lifestyle?

Patient: No, everything has been quite stable.

Doctor: We'll check your weight, height, and blood pressure. I'll also listen to your heart and lungs.

Patient: Will I need any blood tests?

Doctor: Yes, we'll do blood tests to check your cholesterol and sugar levels.

Patient: Should I do anything particular after the exam?

Doctor: Just maintain a healthy lifestyle and follow any specific recommendations that may arise from the exam.

Comprehension Questions

1. **What is the purpose of the visit?**
   a. Vision review
   b. Annual physical exam
   c. Consultation for pain
   d. Hearing check-up

2. **What will the doctor check during the exam?**
   a. Only blood pressure
   b. Stress levels
   c. Weight, height, blood pressure, heart, and lungs
   d. Family history

3. **What additional tests will the doctor order?**
   a. Blood tests for cholesterol and sugar
   b. MRI
   c. Electrocardiogram
   d. Allergy tests

Answers

1. **b)** Examen físico anual - Annual physical exam
2. **c)** Peso, altura, presión arterial, corazón y pulmones - Weight, height, blood pressure, heart, and lungs
3. **a)** Análisis de sangre para colesterol y glucosa - Blood tests for cholesterol and sugar

Revisión de la presión arterial - Blood Pressure Check

Doctor: Buenas tardes. Vamos a revisar tu presión arterial. ¿Has sentido mareos o algo inusual últimamente?

Paciente: Buenas tardes, doctor. No realmente, pero a veces tengo dolores de cabeza leves.

Doctor: Los dolores de cabeza pueden estar relacionados. Vamos a ver cómo está tu presión. ¿Haces ejercicio regularmente?

Paciente: Intento caminar a menudo.

Doctor: Eso es bueno. Caminar ayuda a mantener la presión normal. Vamos a tomar tu presión ahora. Solo relájate.

Preguntas de comprensión

1. **¿Cuál es el motivo de consulta del paciente?**
   a. Control de peso
   b. Revisión de la presión arterial
   c. Revisión de la audición
   d. Examen de la vista

2. **¿Qué síntoma menciona el paciente?**
   a. Dolores de cabeza
   b. Pérdida de apetito
   c. Dificultad para respirar
   d. Cansancio

3. **¿Qué recomendaciones da el doctor para mantener una presión arterial saludable?**
   a. Medicamento especial
   b. Dieta baja en sal y ejercicio
   c. Beber más agua
   d. Descansar más

Dialogue 34:
Blood Pressure Check - Revisión de la presión arterial

Doctor: Good afternoon. We're going to check your blood pressure. Have you felt dizzy or anything unusual lately?

Patient: Good afternoon, Doctor. Not really, but I sometimes have mild headaches.

Doctor: Headaches can be related. Let's see what your blood pressure is. Do you exercise regularly?

Patient: I try to walk often.

Doctor: That's good. Walking helps to keep the pressure normal. Let's take your pressure now. Just relax.

Comprehension Questions

1. **What is the reason for the patient's visit?**
   a. Weight control
   b. Blood pressure check
   c. Hearing check-up
   d. Vision exam

2. **What symptom does the patient mention?**
   a. Headaches
   b. Loss of appetite
   c. Difficulty breathing
   d. Tiredness

3. **What recommendations does the doctor give for maintaining healthy blood pressure?**
   a. Special medication
   b. Low-salt diet and exercise
   c. Drink more water
   d. Rest more

Answers

1. **b)** Revisión de la presión arterial - Blood pressure check
2. **a)** Dolores de cabeza - Headaches
3. **b)** Dieta baja en sal y ejercicio - Low-salt diet and exercise

Revisión del nivel de colesterol - Cholesterol Level Check

Doctor: Hola, hoy revisaremos tus niveles de colesterol. ¿Recuerdas cuándo fue tu última prueba?

Paciente: Hola, doctor. Fue hace aproximadamente un año.

Doctor: ¿Hay casos de colesterol alto en tu familia?

Paciente: Sí, mi padre tuvo problemas con eso.

Doctor: Ya veo. ¿Cómo es tu alimentación habitual? ¿Sueles consumir muchas grasas saturadas?

Paciente: Intento comer bien, pero a veces recurro a la comida rápida.

Doctor: Es clave tener una dieta balanceada. Vamos a analizar tu sangre para ver tu nivel de colesterol.

Paciente: ¿Qué puedo hacer para mantener mi colesterol bajo control?

Doctor: Incrementar la actividad física y comer más frutas, verduras y alimentos bajos en grasas saturadas son pasos importantes y muy útiles.

Preguntas de comprensión

1. **¿Qué prueba se realizará al paciente?**
   a. Prueba de glucosa
   b. Revisión del nivel de colesterol
   c. Revisión de la presión arterial
   d. Prueba de audición

2. **¿Qué antecedente familiar menciona el paciente?**
   a. Diabetes
   b. Hipertensión
   c. Colesterol alto
   d. Artritis

3. **¿Qué consejos da el doctor para mejorar el colesterol?**
   a. Medicamento
   b. Más ejercicio y una dieta balanceada
   c. Evitar salir
   d. Dormir más horas

Cholesterol Level Check -
Revisión del nivel de colesterol

Doctor: Hello, today we'll check your cholesterol levels. Do you remember when you last had it tested?

Patient: Hello, Doctor. It was about a year ago.

Doctor: Any family history of high cholesterol?

Patient: Yes, my father had issues with it.

Doctor: I see. What does your usual diet look like? Do you consume a lot of saturated fats?

Patient: I try to eat healthily, but sometimes I go for fast food.

Doctor: It's important to maintain a balanced diet. We'll take a blood sample to check your cholesterol level.

Patient: What can I do to keep my cholesterol in check?

Doctor: Increasing physical activity and eating more fruits, vegetables, and low-fat foods are key steps.

Comprehension Questions

1. **What test will be performed on the patient?**
   a. Glucose test
   b. Cholesterol level check
   c. Blood pressure examination
   d. Hearing test

2. **What family history does the patient mention?**
   a. Diabetes
   b. Hypertension
   c. High cholesterol
   d. Arthritis

3. **What advice does the doctor give to improve cholesterol?**
   a. Medication
   b. More exercise and a balanced diet
   c. Avoid going out
   d. Sleep more hours

Answers

1. **b)** Revisión del nivel de colesterol - Cholesterol level check
2. **c)** Colesterol alto - High cholesterol
3. **b)** Más ejercicio y una dieta balanceada - More exercise and a balanced diet

Diagnostic Conversations:
Explaining Tests and Results, Follow-Up Care

Clear explanations of diagnostic tests and results are critical for patient understanding and care continuity. This series of dialogues will equip you with the language needed to discuss MRI findings, blood test specifics, and X-ray results. You'll gain the skills to not only relay information accurately but also to handle follow-up care discussions, ensuring patients are fully informed and prepared for the next steps in their healthcare journey.

Discusión de resultados de resonancia magnética - Discussing MRI Results

Doctor: Buenas tardes. He revisado los resultados de tu resonancia magnética y quisiera hablar contigo sobre ellos.

Paciente: Buenas tardes, doctor. ¿Hay algo de qué preocuparme?

Doctor: Los resultados indican una inflamación leve en la rodilla. ¿Has sentido algún dolor o molestia al moverte?

Paciente: Sí, me duele un poco al caminar y al subir escaleras.

Doctor: Entiendo, eso explica los resultados. Vamos a empezar un tratamiento antiinflamatorio y considerar fisioterapia para aliviar el dolor.

Paciente: ¿Será necesario hacerme otra resonancia en el futuro?

Doctor: Vamos a ver cómo evoluciona con el tratamiento y decidiremos si es necesario. Te daremos seguimiento con consultas regulares.

Paciente: ¿Hay algo más que pueda hacer por mi cuenta para mejorar?

Doctor: Sí, te aconsejo descansar la rodilla y evitar actividades que puedan agravar el dolor. También te daré algunas recomendaciones para cuidarla en casa.

Preguntas de comprensión

1. **¿Qué muestra la resonancia magnética del paciente?**
   a. Un hueso roto
   b. Inflamación en la rodilla
   c. Una infección
   d. Problemas en el corazón

2. **¿Qué tratamiento propone el doctor?**
   a. Cirugía inmediata
   b. Tratamiento antiinflamatorio y fisioterapia
   c. Reposo absoluto
   d. Cambio de dieta

3. **¿Qué recomienda el doctor para el cuidado de la rodilla?**
   a. Evitar el reposo
   b. Hacer ejercicios intensos
   c. Descansar la rodilla y evitar ciertas actividades
   d. Tomar analgésicos regularmente

Discussing MRI Results - Discusión de resultados de resonancia magnética

Doctor: Good afternoon. I've reviewed your MRI results and I'd like to discuss them with you.

Patient: Good afternoon, Doctor. Is there anything to be concerned about?

Doctor: The results show mild inflammation in your knee. Have you been experiencing any pain or discomfort when moving?

Patient: Yes, it hurts a bit when I walk and go up stairs.

Doctor: I see, that explains the results. We'll start an anti-inflammatory treatment and consider physiotherapy to relieve the pain.

Patient: Will I need another MRI in the future?

Doctor: We'll see how it evolves with the treatment and then decide if it's necessary. We'll keep track with regular follow-ups.

Patient: Is there anything else I can do myself to improve?

Doctor: Yes, I advise you to rest your knee and avoid activities that might worsen the pain. I'll also give you some recommendations to take care of it at home.

Comprehension Questions

1. **What does the patient's MRI show?**
   - a. A broken bone
   - b. Inflammation in the knee
   - c. An infection
   - d. Heart problems

2. **What treatment does the doctor propose?**
   - a. Immediate surgery
   - b. Anti-inflammatory treatment and physiotherapy
   - c. Complete rest
   - d. Diet change

3. **What does the doctor recommend for knee care?**
   - a. Avoid resting
   - b. Do intense exercises
   - c. Rest the knee and avoid certain activities
   - d. Take painkillers regularly

Answers

1. **b)** Inflamación en la rodilla - Inflammation in the knee
2. **b)** Tratamiento antiinflamatorio y fisioterapia - Anti-inflammatory treatment and physiotherapy
3. **c)** Descansar la rodilla y evitar ciertas actividades - Rest the knee and avoid certain activities

Explicación de un análisis de sangre - Explaining a Blood Test

Doctor: Hola, vamos a hablar sobre los resultados de tu análisis de sangre.

Paciente: Hola, doctor. ¿Debería estar preocupado?

Doctor: No hay motivos de alarma. Tus resultados en general son buenos, pero tus niveles de azúcar en sangre están ligeramente elevados.

Paciente: ¿Eso significa que podría tener diabetes?

Doctor: No directamente, pero debemos prestar atención. ¿Alguien en tu familia tiene diabetes?

Paciente: Sí, mi madre.

Doctor: Entonces es importante controlar tu dieta y aumentar tu actividad física. Te daré algunas recomendaciones.

Paciente: ¿Cuándo debería hacerme otro análisis?

Doctor: Vamos a repetirlo en unos meses para verificar la evolución.

Preguntas de comprensión

1. **¿Qué se está discutiendo en la consulta?**
   a. Resultados de una resonancia magnética
   b. Resultados de una prueba de visión
   c. Resultados de un análisis de sangre
   d. Resultados de una prueba de audición

2. **¿Qué indicador anormal encontraron en la sangre del paciente?**
   a. Colesterol alto
   b. Bajo nivel de hierro
   c. Niveles elevados de azúcar
   d. Infección

3. **¿Qué recomienda el doctor para controlar el indicador anormal?**
   a. Medicamento inmediato
   b. Cambios en la dieta y más ejercicio
   c. Reposo en cama
   d. Cirugía

Explaining a Blood Test - Explicación de un análisis de sangre

Doctor: Hello, today we will discuss your blood test results.

Patient: Hello, Doctor. Is there anything concerning?

Doctor: Your results are mostly good, but your blood sugar levels are a bit high.

Patient: Does that mean I could have diabetes?

Doctor: Not necessarily, but it's something we need to monitor. Does diabetes run in your family?

Patient: Yes, my mother has it.

Doctor: It's vital to monitor your diet and increase physical activity. I'll give you some guidance.

Patient: When should I have another test?

Doctor: We'll do a follow-up test in a few months to track the changes.

Comprehension Questions

1. **What is discussed in the consultation?**
   a. MRI results
   b. Vision test results
   c. Blood test results
   d. Hearing test results

2. **What abnormal indicator was found in the patient's blood?**
   a. High cholesterol
   b. Low iron level
   c. Elevated sugar levels
   d. Infection

3. **What does the doctor recommend to control the abnormal indicator?**
   a. Immediate medication
   b. Dietary changes and more exercise
   c. Bed rest
   d. Surgery

Answers

1. **c)** Resultados de un análisis de sangre - Blood test results
2. **c)** Niveles elevados de azúcar - Elevated sugar levels
3. **b)** Cambios en la dieta y más ejercicio - Dietary changes and more exercise

Diálogo 38: Discusión de resultados de rayos X - Discussing X-ray Results

Doctor: Hola, he revisado tus rayos X y quiero hablar sobre los resultados.

Paciente: Hola, doctor. ¿Hay algo preocupante en los rayos X?

Doctor: La radiografía muestra una pequeña fractura en tu tobillo.

Paciente: ¿Eso explica el dolor y la dificultad para caminar que he tenido?

Doctor: Sí, es probablemente la causa. Necesitaremos inmovilizar tu tobillo para que se repare correctamente.

Paciente: ¿Cuánto tiempo tardará en curarse?

Doctor: Las fracturas pequeñas suelen tardar unas seis semanas.

Paciente: ¿Y después voy a necesitar fisioterapia?

Doctor: Sí, será necesario para recuperar la movilidad y fortalecer el tobillo.

Preguntas de comprensión

1. **¿Qué mostraron los rayos X del paciente?**
   a. Una infección pulmonar
   b. Una fractura en el tobillo
   c. Artritis en la rodilla
   d. Problemas cardíacos

2. **¿Qué tratamiento se necesita para la fractura?**
   a. Inmovilización del tobillo
   b. Antibióticos
   c. Cirugía inmediata
   d. Cambio de dieta

3. **¿Qué se recomienda después de la sanación de la fractura?**
   a. Reposo prolongado
   b. Fisioterapia
   c. Evitar el ejercicio
   d. Continuar con medicamento

Dialogue 38:
Discussing X-ray Results -
Discusión de resultados de rayos X

Doctor: Hello, I've reviewed your X-rays and want to discuss the results.

Patient: Hello, Doctor. Is there something wrong in the X-rays?

Doctor: The X-rays show that you have a small fracture in your ankle.

Patient: Does that explain why I've been having pain and difficulty walking?

Doctor: Yes, it's likely the cause. We'll need to immobilize your ankle for proper healing.

Patient: How long will the healing take?

Doctor: Small fractures typically heal in about six weeks.

Patient: Will I require physiotherapy afterward?

Doctor: Yes, it will be necessary to regain mobility and strengthen the ankle.

Comprehension Questions

1. **What did the patient's X-rays show?**
   a. A lung infection
   b. A fracture in the ankle
   c. Arthritis in the knee
   d. Heart problems

2. **What treatment is needed for the fracture?**
   a. Immobilization of the ankle
   b. Antibiotics
   c. Immediate surgery
   d. Diet change

3. **What is recommended after the fracture heals?**
   a. Prolonged rest
   b. Physiotherapy
   c. Avoid exercise
   d. Continue with medication

Answers

1. **b)** Una fractura en el tobillo - A fracture in the ankle
2. **a)** Inmovilización del tobillo - Immobilization of the ankle
3. **b)** Fisioterapia - Physiotherapy

Pharmacy Interactions:
Medication Instructions, Managing Side Effects

Pharmacy interactions are pivotal moments for ensuring patient safety and treatment efficacy. This dialogue series focuses on the intricacies of prescribing medication, explaining dosage instructions, and discussing potential side effects. You'll navigate conversations around hypertension treatments, antibiotic usage, and pain management, providing you with the vocabulary to offer clear guidance and support patients in their medication regimen.

Diálogo 39: Tratamiento de la hipertensión - Medication for Hypertension

Farmacéutico: Buenos días. Aquí tienes tu medicamento para la hipertensión. Vamos a hablar sobre cómo tomarlo.

Paciente: Buenos días. Estoy un poco preocupado. ¿Cómo debo hacerlo?

Farmacéutico: Entiendo tu preocupación. Es importante tomar una pastilla al día, preferentemente en la mañana.

Paciente: ¿Y hay efectos secundarios?

Farmacéutico: Al principio, puedes sentir algo de mareo. Si eso sucede, es mejor no conducir.

Paciente: ¿Qué hago si olvido tomarla algún día?

Farmacéutico: Si te acuerdas el mismo día, tómala tan pronto como puedas. Si no, sigue con la dosis habitual al día siguiente.

Paciente: ¿Debería cambiar algo en mi alimentación?

Farmacéutico: Sí, te ayudaría seguir una dieta baja en sal. Además, el ejercicio regular es muy beneficioso.

Preguntas de comprensión

1. **¿Para qué es el medicamento que el paciente debe tomar?**
   a. Diabetes
   b. Hipertensión
   c. Colesterol alto
   d. Artritis

2. **¿Qué consejo da el farmacéutico sobre cuándo tomar la medicación?**
   a. Con cada comida
   b. Antes de dormir
   c. Una vez al día por la mañana
   d. Sólo cuando se sienta mal

3. **¿Qué recomendación dietética hace el farmacéutico?**
   a. Evitar el azúcar
   b. Comer más proteínas
   c. Bajar el consumo de sal
   d. Aumentar los carbohidratos

Medication for Hypertension - Tratamiento de la hipertensión

Pharmacist: Good morning. Here's your medication for hypertension. Let's discuss how to take it.

Patient: Good morning. I'm a bit worried. How should I do it?

Pharmacist: I understand your concern. It's important to take one pill daily, preferably in the morning.

Patient: What about side effects?

Pharmacist: Initially, you might experience some dizziness. If that happens, avoid driving.

Patient: What if I forget to take it one day?

Pharmacist: If you remember the same day, take it as soon as possible. Otherwise, just continue with your usual dose the next day.

Patient: Should I change anything in my diet?

Pharmacist: Yes, following a low-salt diet would be helpful. Regular exercise is also very beneficial.

Comprehension Questions

1. **What is the patient's medication for?**
   a. Diabetes
   b. Hypertension
   c. High cholesterol
   d. Arthritis

2. **What advice does the pharmacist give about when to take the medication?**
   a. With each meal
   b. Before sleeping
   c. Once a day in the morning
   d. Only when feeling unwell

3. **What dietary recommendation does the pharmacist make?**
   a. Avoid sugar
   b. Eat more protein
   c. Lower salt intake
   d. Increase carbohydrates

Answers

1. **b)** Hipertensión - Hypertension
2. **c)** Una vez al día por la mañana - Once a day in the morning
3. **c)** Bajar el consumo de sal - Lower salt intake

Indicaciones para antibióticos - Antibiotics Instructions

Farmacéutico: Hola, voy a darte las indicaciones para tus antibióticos.

Paciente: Hola, gracias. ¿Cómo debo tomarlos?

Farmacéutico: Toma una pastilla cada ocho horas, con o sin alimentos.

Paciente: ¿Qué hago si olvido una dosis?

Farmacéutico: En cuanto te des cuenta, tómala lo antes posible. No tomes dos dosis al mismo tiempo.

Paciente: ¿Y hay efectos secundarios?

Farmacéutico: Es posible que sientas náuseas o diarrea. Bebe bastante agua.

Paciente: ¿Debo completar todo el tratamiento?

Farmacéutico: Sí, es crucial completar todo el tratamiento de antibióticos para prevenir la resistencia a los mismos y asegurar su eficacia. Aunque te sientas mejor, es importante terminarlos.

Preguntas de comprensión

1. **¿Para qué es el medicamento que el paciente recibirá?**
   a. Para la presión arterial
   b. Para el colesterol
   c. Para una infección
   d. Para el dolor

2. **¿Qué debe hacer el paciente si se salta una dosis?**
   a. Tomar una dosis doble la próxima vez
   b. Tomar la dosis olvidada lo antes posible
   c. Ignorar la dosis olvidada y continuar
   d. Llamar al médico inmediatamente

3. **¿Cuál es la importancia de terminar el tratamiento de antibióticos?**
   a. Evitar efectos secundarios
   b. Prevenir resistencia a los antibióticos
   c. Reducir el riesgo de alergias
   d. Mantener el medicamento efectivo

Pharmacist: Hello, I'm going to give you instructions for taking these antibiotics.

Patient: Hello, thank you. How should I take them?

Pharmacist: Take one pill every eight hours, with or without food.

Patient: What if I miss a dose?

Pharmacist: Once you realize, take it as soon as possible. Do not take two doses at the same time.

Patient: Are there any side effects?

Pharmacist: You may experience nausea or diarrhea. Make sure to drink plenty of water.

Patient: Should I complete the entire course of antibiotics?

Pharmacist: Yes, it's crucial to complete the entire course of antibiotics to prevent antibiotic resistance and ensure their effectiveness. Even if you feel better, it's important to finish them.

Comprehension Questions

1. **What is the patient's medication for?**
   a. Blood pressure
   b. Cholesterol
   c. An infection
   d. Pain

2. **What should the patient do if they miss a dose?**
   a. Take a double dose next time
   b. Take the missed dose as soon as possible
   c. Skip the missed dose and continue
   d. Call the doctor immediately

3. **Why is it important to complete the antibiotic course?**
   a. To avoid side effects
   b. To prevent antibiotic resistance
   c. To reduce the risk of allergies
   d. To keep the medication effective

Answers

1. **c)** Para una infección - For an infection
2. **b)** Tomar la dosis olvidada lo antes posible - Take the missed dose as soon as possible
3. **b)** Prevenir resistencia a los antibióticos - To prevent antibiotic resistance

Tratamiento del dolor - Pain Medication

Farmacéutico: Hola, aquí tienes tu medicamento para el dolor. Es importante tomarlo correctamente.

Paciente: Hola, gracias. ¿Cuál es la mejor forma de tomarlo?

Farmacéutico: Toma una pastilla cada seis horas. Es mejor si la tomas con comida para cuidar tu estómago.

Paciente: ¿Y qué pasa si me olvido de tomarla?

Farmacéutico: Si te olvidas, tómala tan pronto como recuerdes, pero nunca tomes dos dosis juntas.

Paciente: De acuerdo. ¿Esta medicina tiene efectos secundarios?

Farmacéutico: Podrías sentirte un poco somnoliento o mareado. Ten cuidado, especialmente si vas a conducir.

Paciente: Gracias por la información. ¿Hay algo más que deba saber?

Farmacéutico: Sí, si el dolor no mejora o empeora, es importante que hables con tu médico.

Preguntas de comprensión

1. **¿Para qué es el medicamento que el farmacéutico está explicando?**
   a. Hipertensión
   b. Diabetes
   c. Dolor
   d. Insomnio

2. **¿Qué recomendación da el farmacéutico si el dolor no mejora?**
   a. Tomar más medicamento
   b. Consultar al médico
   c. Cambiar la dieta
   d. Hacer ejercicio

3. **¿Cuál es un posible efecto secundario del medicamento?**
   a. Somnolencia o mareos
   b. Aumento de peso
   c. Visión borrosa
   d. Aumento del apetito

Pain Medication - Tratamiento del dolor

Pharmacist: Hello, here's your pain medication. It's important to take it correctly.

Patient: Hello, thank you. What's the best way to take it?

Pharmacist: Take one pill every six hours. It's better to take it with food to protect your stomach.

Patient: And what if I forget to take it?

Pharmacist: If you forget, take it as soon as you remember, but never take two doses together.

Patient: I see. Does this medicine have side effects?

Pharmacist: You might feel a bit drowsy or dizzy. Be careful, especially if you're going to drive.

Patient: Thanks for the information. Is there anything else I should know?

Pharmacist: Yes, if the pain doesn't improve or gets worse, it's important to talk to your doctor.

Comprehension Questions

1. **What is the medication the pharmacist is explaining?**
   - a. Hypertension
   - b. Diabetes
   - c. Pain
   - d. Insomnia

2. **What does the pharmacist recommend if the pain does not improve?**
   - a. Take more medication
   - b. Consult the doctor
   - c. Change the diet
   - d. Exercise

3. **What is a possible side effect of the medication?**
   - a. Drowsiness or dizziness
   - b. Weight gain
   - c. Blurred vision
   - d. Increased appetite

Answers

1. **c)** Dolor - Pain
2. **b)** Consultar al médico - Consult the doctor
3. **a)** Somnolencia o mareos - Drowsiness or dizziness

Nutritional Counseling:
Dietary Advice for Health Conditions

Nutritional counseling plays a key role in managing and preventing various health conditions. Through these dialogues, you'll delve into providing dietary advice tailored to diabetes management, weight loss strategies, and heart-healthy eating habits. Learn how to communicate effectively about nutrition, empowering your patients to make informed choices that positively impact their health.

Consejos dietéticos para la diabetes - Dietary Advice for Diabetes

Nutricionista: Buenas tardes. Vamos a hablar sobre tu dieta para controlar la diabetes.

Paciente: Buenas tardes. ¿Qué debería comer?

Nutricionista: Es importante equilibrar los carbohidratos con proteínas y grasas saludables. Debes evitar el azúcar y los carbohidratos refinados.

Paciente: ¿Puedo comer fruta?

Nutricionista: Sí, pero con moderación, especialmente las frutas con alto contenido de azúcar.

Paciente: ¿Y bocadillos?

Nutricionista: Opta por bocadillos bajos en carbohidratos, como vegetales crudos o nueces.

Paciente: ¿Necesito contar los carbohidratos?

Nutricionista: Sí, te ayudará a controlar tus niveles de azúcar en sangre. Te enseñaré cómo hacerlo.

Preguntas de comprensión

1. **¿Qué tema se está discutiendo en la consulta?**
   a. Consejos para bajar de peso
   b. Dieta para la hipertensión
   c. Consejos dietéticos para la diabetes
   d. Alimentación para la salud cardíaca

2. **¿Qué debe limitar el paciente en su dieta?**
   a. Grasas
   b. Azúcares y carbohidratos refinados
   c. Proteínas
   d. Lácteos

3. **¿Qué recomienda el nutricionista para los bocadillos?**
   a. Evitarlos completamente
   b. Sólo frutas
   c. Bocadillos bajos en carbohidratos
   d. Alimentos ricos en fibra

Dietary Advice for Diabetes - Consejos dietéticos para la diabetes

Nutritionist: Good afternoon. Let's talk about your diet to manage diabetes.

Patient: Good afternoon. What should I eat?

Nutritionist: It's important to balance carbohydrates with proteins and healthy fats. You should avoid sugar and refined carbohydrates.

Patient: Can I eat fruit?

Nutritionist: Yes, but in moderation, especially fruits high in sugar.

Patient: What about snacks?

Nutritionist: Choose low-carbohydrate snacks like raw vegetables or nuts.

Patient: Do I need to count carbohydrates?

Nutritionist: Yes, it will help you control your blood sugar levels. I'll teach you how to do it.

Comprehension Questions

1. **What topic is being discussed in the consultation?**
   a. Advice for weight loss
   b. Diet for hypertension
   c. Dietary advice for diabetes
   d. Nutrition for heart health

2. **What should the patient limit in their diet?**
   a. Fats
   b. Sugars and refined carbohydrates
   c. Proteins
   d. Dairy

3. **What does the nutritionist recommend for snacks?**
   a. Avoid them completely
   b. Only fruits
   c. Low-carbohydrate snacks
   d. High-fiber foods

Answers

1. **c)** Consejos dietéticos para la diabetes - Dietary advice for diabetes
2. **b)** Azúcares y carbohidratos refinados - Sugars and refined carbohydrates
3. **c)** Bocadillos bajos en carbohidratos - Low-carbohydrate snacks

Dieta para la pérdida de peso - Weight Loss Diet

Nutricionista: Hola, veo que quieres mejorar tu alimentación para perder peso. ¿Cómo sueles comer actualmente?

Paciente: Hola, sí, necesito ayuda. Normalmente como rápido y no siempre de manera saludable.

Nutricionista: Entiendo, es un buen primer paso reconocerlo. Lo ideal es elegir alimentos nutritivos y balanceados.

Paciente: ¿Cómo debería organizar mis comidas?

Nutricionista: Te recomiendo tres comidas principales y dos bocadillos saludables al día para activar tu metabolismo.

Paciente: ¿Qué puedo comer como bocadillo?

Nutricionista: Algunas frutas, yogur natural, o un puñado de frutos secos son excelentes opciones.

Paciente: ¿El ejercicio también es importante?

Nutricionista: Claro, el ejercicio regular te ayudará a perder peso de manera más efectiva. Te recomiendo combinar ejercicios de cardio con ejercicios de fuerza.

Preguntas de comprensión

1. **¿Cuál es el objetivo del paciente en la consulta?**
   a. Aprender a cocinar
   b. Bajar la presión arterial
   c. Perder peso
   d. Mejorar la digestión

2. **¿Qué cambio en la dieta sugiere el nutricionista?**
   a. Comer sólo alimentos orgánicos
   b. Más frutas, verduras, y proteínas magras
   c. Eliminar todos los carbohidratos
   d. Sólo beber batidos

3. **¿Qué importancia tiene el ejercicio según el nutricionista?**
   a. No es necesario para perder peso
   b. Es crucial y debe incluir cardio y fuerza
   c. Sólo yoga y meditación
   d. Ejercicio ligero una vez a la semana

Weight Loss Diet - Dieta para la pérdida de peso

Nutritionist: Hello, I see you're looking to improve your diet for weight loss. What is your typical diet like?

Patient: Hello, yes, I need guidance. I usually eat fast and not always healthily.

Nutritionist: It's good to recognize that as a first step. It's best to choose nutritious and balanced foods.

Patient: How should I organize my meals?

Nutritionist: I recommend three main meals and two healthy snacks a day to keep your metabolism active.

Patient: What can I have for a snack?

Nutritionist: Fruits, natural yogurt, or a handful of nuts are great choices.

Patient: Is exercise also important?

Nutritionist: Absolutely, regular exercise will help you lose weight more effectively. I suggest combining cardio with some strength training.

Comprehension Questions

1. **What is the patient's goal in the consultation?**
   a. Learn to cook
   b. Lower blood pressure
   c. Lose weight
   d. Improve digestion

2. **What dietary change does the nutritionist suggest?**
   a. Eat only organic foods
   b. More fruits, vegetables, and lean proteins
   c. Eliminate all carbohydrates
   d. Only drink shakes

3. **How important is exercise according to the nutritionist?**
   a. Not necessary for weight loss
   b. Crucial and should include cardio and strength
   c. Only yoga and meditation
   d. Light exercise once a week

Answers

1. **c)** Perder peso - Lose weight
2. **b)** Más frutas, verduras, y proteínas magras - More fruits, vegetables, and lean proteins
3. **b)** Es crucial y debe incluir cardio y fuerza - Crucial and should include cardio and strength

Diálogo 44:
Dieta para la salud cardíaca - Heart-Healthy Diet

Nutricionista: Hola, hoy vamos a enfocarnos en una dieta saludable para tu corazón. ¿Qué sueles comer habitualmente?

Paciente: Hola. Mi dieta no es muy buena. Como muchos alimentos procesados y grasosos.

Nutritionist: Para proteger tu corazón, es importante comer alimentos bajos en grasas saturadas y trans. Incluye más frutas, verduras y granos enteros.

Paciente: ¿Debo evitar las carnes rojas?

Nutricionista: No necesariamente, pero elige cortes magros y limita su consumo. Prefiere pescado, pollo y legumbres.

Paciente: ¿Qué tipo de grasas son saludables?

Nutricionista: Las grasas monoinsaturadas y poliinsaturadas son buenas. Las encuentras en el aceite de oliva, nueces y pescado.

Paciente: ¿Y en cuanto a los lácteos?

Nutricionista: Opta por versiones bajas en grasa o desnatadas. También es importante limitar el consumo de sal y azúcar.

Preguntas de comprensión

1. **¿Cuál es el enfoque de la dieta que se discute?**
   a. Dieta para perder peso
   b. Dieta para la diabetes
   c. Dieta para la salud cardíaca
   d. Dieta baja en carbohidratos

2. **¿Qué debe limitar el paciente en su dieta según el nutricionista?**
   a. Todas las carnes
   b. Grasas saturadas y trans
   c. Todos los lácteos
   d. El pan y los cereales

3. **¿Qué recomienda el nutricionista sobre el consumo de carnes?**
   a. Evitar completamente
   b. Sólo carnes rojas
   c. Cortes magros y limitar su consumo
   d. Sólo carnes procesadas

Dialogue 44:
Heart-Healthy Diet - Dieta para la salud cardíaca

Nutritionist: Hello, today we'll focus on a heart-healthy diet. What do you usually eat?

Patient: Hello. My diet isn't very good. I eat a lot of processed and fatty foods.

Nutritionist: To protect your heart, it's important to eat foods low in saturated and trans fats. Include more fruits, vegetables, and whole grains.

Patient: Should I avoid red meat?

Nutritionist: Not necessarily, but choose lean cuts and limit its consumption. Prefer fish, chicken, and legumes.

Patient: What kinds of fats are healthy?

Nutritionist: Monounsaturated and polyunsaturated fats are good. You find them in olive oil, nuts, and fish.

Patient: What about dairy products?

Nutritionist: Choose low-fat or non-fat versions. It's also important to limit your intake of salt and sugar.

Comprehension Questions

1. **What is the focus of the diet being discussed?**
   a. Diet for weight loss
   b. Diet for diabetes
   c. Heart-healthy diet
   d. Low-carb diet

2. **What should the patient limit in their diet according to the nutritionist?**
   a. All meats
   b. Saturated and trans fats
   c. All dairy
   d. Bread and cereals

3. **What does the nutritionist recommend about meat consumption?**
   a. Avoid completely
   b. Only red meats
   c. Lean cuts and limit consumption
   d. Only processed meats

Answers

1. **c)** Dieta para la salud cardíaca - Heart-healthy diet
2. **b)** Grasas saturadas y trans - Saturated and trans fats
3. **c)** Cortes magros y limitar su consumo - Lean cuts and limit consumption

Post-Operative Care:
Post-Surgery Care, Wound Care, Recovery Instructions

Effective post-operative care is crucial for a patient's recovery and long-term health. This set of dialogues covers essential aspects of post-surgery communication, including providing instructions after minor and major surgeries, managing wound care, and guiding patients through their recovery process. You'll acquire the language skills necessary to support patients post-operation, ensuring they receive the care and information needed for a smooth and safe recovery.

Diálogo 45: Indicaciones postoperatorias en cirugía menor - Instructions After Minor Surgery

Enfermero: Hola, te voy a dar algunas indicaciones postoperatorias para tu cirugía menor.

Paciente: Hola, gracias. ¿Qué debo hacer cuando llegue a casa?

Enfermero: Debes descansar y evitar esfuerzos físicos por unos días.

Paciente: ¿Puedo ducharme normalmente?

Enfermero: Espera al menos 24 horas antes de ducharte y evita mojar directamente la herida.

Paciente: ¿Qué hago si siento dolor?

Enfermero: Puedes tomar el analgésico recetado según las indicaciones. Si el dolor es muy intenso, contacta a tu médico.

Paciente: ¿Cuándo debo regresar para una revisión?

Enfermero: Tendremos una cita de seguimiento en una semana para revisar tu progreso.

Paciente: ¿Hay algo más que deba saber?

Enfermero: Sigue las instrucciones sobre el medicamento y el cuidado de la herida. Llámanos si tienes alguna duda.

Preguntas de comprensión

1. **¿Cuál es el propósito de las indicaciones dadas al paciente?**
   a. Cuidado de la diabetes
   b. Recuperación de una cirugía menor
   c. Manejo del estrés
   d. Preparación para un examen médico

2. **¿Qué debe evitar el paciente después de la cirugía?**
   a. Comer alimentos sólidos
   b. Hacer esfuerzos físicos
   c. Beber líquidos
   d. Tomar medicamentos

3. **¿Cuándo puede el paciente ducharse después de la cirugía?**
   a. Inmediatamente después
   b. En una semana
   c. Cuando se retiren los puntos
   d. Después de 24 horas

Instructions After Minor Surgery -
Indicaciones postoperatorias en cirugía menor

Nurse: Hello, I'm going to give you some postoperative instructions after your minor surgery.

Patient: Hello, thank you. What should I do when I get home?

Nurse: You should rest and avoid physical exertion for a few days.

Patient: Can I shower normally?

Nurse: Wait at least 24 hours before showering and avoid wetting the wound directly.

Patient: What should I do if I feel pain?

Nurse: You can take the prescribed painkiller as directed. If the pain is very intense, contact your doctor.

Patient: When should I come back for a check-up?

Nurse: We have a follow-up appointment in a week to check your progress.

Patient: Is there anything else I should know?

Nurse: Follow the instructions for medication and wound care. Call if you have questions or concerns.

Comprehension Questions

1. **What is the purpose of the instructions given to the patient?**
   a. Diabetes care
   b. Recovery from minor surgery
   c. Stress management
   d. Preparation for a medical exam

2. **What should the patient avoid after surgery?**
   a. Eating solid foods
   b. Physical exertion
   c. Drinking liquids
   d. Taking medication

3. **When can the patient shower after the surgery?**
   a. Immediately afterward
   b. In a week
   c. When the stitches are removed
   d. After 24 hours

Answers

1. **b)** Recuperación de una cirugía menor - Recovery from minor surgery
2. **b)** Hacer esfuerzos físicos - Physical exertion
3. **d)** Después de 24 horas - After 24 hours

Cuidado de la herida quirúrgica - Wound Care

Enfermero: Hola, voy a explicarte cómo cuidar tu herida para que se cure correctamente.

Paciente: Hola, ¿qué debo hacer?

Enfermero: Primero, mantén la herida limpia y seca. Cambia el vendaje según las indicaciones.

Paciente: ¿Puedo mojar la herida cuando me ducho?

Enfermero: Trata de evitar mojarla directamente. Puedes cubrirla con un plástico impermeable.

Paciente: ¿Qué signos vería en caso de infección?

Enfermero: Si la herida se enrojece, le sale pus, o si sientes un aumento del dolor, avísanos de inmediato.

Paciente: ¿Debo usar alguna crema o pomada?

Enfermero: Sí, aplicar una pomada antibiótica puede ser recomendable. Te indicaré cuál usar.

Paciente: ¿Cuánto tiempo tardará en curarse?

Enfermero: Depende del tipo y tamaño de la herida, pero te daremos un estimado en tu próxima cita.

Preguntas de comprensión

1. **¿Qué debe hacer el paciente para cuidar la herida?**
   a. Mantenerla caliente y húmeda
   b. Mantenerla limpia y seca
   c. Cubrirla con un vendaje apretado
   d. Aplicar calor directamente

2. **¿Cómo debe el paciente ducharse para proteger la herida?**
   a. Ducharse normalmente
   b. No ducharse hasta que se cure
   c. Cubrir la herida con un plástico
   d. Usar sólo agua fría

3. **¿Qué indicaría una infección en la herida?**
   a. Enrojecimiento y supuración
   b. Menos dolor alrededor de la herida
   c. Cambio de color en el vendaje
   d. Cicatrización rápida

Dialogue 46:
Wound Care - Cuidado de la herida quirúrgica

Nurse: Hello, I'm going to explain how to care for your wound so it heals properly.

Patient: Hello, what should I do?

Nurse: First, keep the wound clean and dry. Change the dressing as directed.

Patient: Can I wet the wound when I shower?

Nurse: Try to avoid wetting it directly. You can cover it with waterproof plastic wrap.

Patient: What signs of infection should I look for?

Nurse: If the wound becomes red, oozes, or if you feel an increase in pain, let us know immediately.

Patient: Should I use any cream or ointment?

Nurse: Yes, applying an antibiotic ointment can be advisable. I'll tell you which one to use.

Patient: How long will it take to heal?

Nurse: It depends on the type and size of the wound, but we'll give you an estimate at your next appointment.

Comprehension Questions

1. **What should the patient do to care for the wound?**
   a. Keep it warm and moist
   b. Keep it clean and dry
   c. Cover it with a tight bandage
   d. Apply direct heat

2. **How should the patient shower to protect the wound?**
   a. Shower normally
   b. Not shower until it heals
   c. Cover the wound with plastic
   d. Use only cold water

3. **What would indicate an infection in the wound?**
   a. Redness and oozing
   b. Less pain around the wound
   c. Change of color in the bandage
   d. Rapid healing

Answers

1. **b)** Mantenerla limpia y seca - Keep it clean and dry
2. **c)** Cubrir la herida con un plástico - Cover the wound with plastic
3. **a)** Enrojecimiento y supuración - Redness and oozing

Recuperación postoperatoria en cirugía mayor – Recovery from Major Surgery

Enfermero: Hola, qué bueno verte. Vamos a cuidarte bien después de la cirugía. ¿Cómo te sientes hoy?

Paciente: Hola, gracias por preguntar. Estoy algo preocupado. ¿Qué debería hacer?

Enfermero: Primero, es muy importante descansar. Evita hacer ejercicios intensos durante unas semanas.

Paciente: ¿Cuándo podré volver a mis actividades habituales?

Enfermero: Cada persona es diferente, pero podrían ser semanas o incluso meses. Te acompañaremos en cada paso de tu recuperación.

Paciente: ¿Qué tipo de alimentos son buenos para mí ahora?

Enfermero: Una dieta balanceada, con muchas proteínas, frutas y verduras te ayudará a recuperarte más rápido.

Paciente: ¿Qué hago si siento mucho dolor?

Enfermero: Te vamos a dar medicinas para el dolor. Si no te alivian, avísanos por favor.

Paciente: ¿Y después necesitaré terapia?

Enfermero: Sí, la terapia es importante. Vamos a planificar sesiones de fisioterapia para ayudarte a recuperarte completamente.

Preguntas de comprensión

1. **¿Qué es esencial para la recuperación después de una cirugía mayor?**
   a. Ejercicio inmediato
   b. Regresar al trabajo lo antes posible
   c. Viajar
   d. Descanso y evitar actividades físicas intensas

2. **¿Qué tipo de dieta debe seguir el paciente?**
   a. Dieta baja en calorías
   b. Dieta líquida
   c. Dieta rica en proteínas y nutrientes
   d. Dieta sin carbohidratos

3. **¿Cuál es el plan para el manejo del dolor postoperatorio?**
   a. No tomar medicamentos
   b. Sólo remedios naturales
   c. Medicamento continuo sin supervisión

d. Analgésicos recetados y
   monitoreo del dolor

Recovery from Major Surgery - Recuperación postoperatoria en cirugía mayor

Nurse: Hello, it's good to see you. We're here to take good care of you after your surgery. How are you feeling today?

Patient: Hello, thank you for asking. I'm a bit worried. What should I do?

Nurse: First, it's very important to rest. Avoid any heavy exercises for a few weeks.

Patient: When can I get back to my usual activities?

Nurse: Everyone is different, but it could be weeks or even months. We will be with you every step of your recovery.

Patient: What kind of food is good for me now?

Nurse: A balanced diet, with lots of proteins, fruits, and vegetables will help you heal faster.

Patient: What if I feel a lot of pain?

Nurse: We will give you pain medication. If they don't relieve your pain, please let us know.

Patient: And afterward, will I need therapy?

Nurse: Yes, therapy is important. We will plan physiotherapy sessions to help you fully recover.

Comprehension Questions

1. **What is essential for recovery after major surgery?**
   a. Immediate exercise
   b. Returning to work as soon as possible
   c. Traveling
   d. Rest and avoiding intense physical activities

2. **What type of diet should the patient follow?**
   a. Low-calorie diet
   b. Liquid diet
   c. Protein and nutrient-rich diet
   d. No-carb diet

3. **What is the plan for postoperative pain management?**
   a. Not taking any medication
   b. Only natural remedies

c. Continuous medication without supervision

d. Prescribed painkillers and monitoring of pain

Answers

1. **d)** Descanso y evitar actividades físicas intensas - Rest and avoiding intense physical activities
2. **c)** Dieta rica en proteínas y nutrientes - Protein and nutrient-rich diet
3. **d)** Analgésicos recetados y monitoreo del dolor - Prescribed painkillers and monitoring of pain

Dermatological Concerns:
Skin Conditions, Allergies, and Treatments

Dermatology involves a wide range of conditions affecting the skin, from common allergies to more specific disorders like eczema and acne. In this series of dialogues, you'll explore how to discuss symptoms, provide advice on managing skin conditions, and explain treatment options. Learn the essential Spanish vocabulary and phrases to help patients understand their dermatological health, ensuring effective communication about care plans and expected outcomes.

Manejo del eczema - Eczema Management

Dermatólogo: Buenos días. Hoy vamos a cuidar tu piel y hablar sobre tu eczema.

Paciente: Buenos días, doctor. ¿Qué puedo hacer para controlar los brotes?

Dermatólogo: Lo más importante es mantener la piel hidratada. Utiliza cremas especiales para pieles sensibles.

Paciente: ¿Hay algo que debería evitar?

Dermatólogo: Evita jabones fuertes y detergentes, pues podrían irritar tu piel.. Y recuerda, no te rasques para no dañarla más.

Paciente: ¿Influye la dieta en el eczema?

Dermatólogo: A veces, ciertos alimentos pueden hacerlo peor. Te ayudaré a identificarlos con un diario de comidas.

Paciente: ¿Y hay tratamientos médicos para el eczema?

Dermatólogo: Sí, hay cremas con corticosteroides que alivian la inflamación. Te mostraré cómo usarlas correctamente.

Preguntas de comprensión

1. **¿Cuál es el enfoque principal para manejar el eczema según el dermatólogo?**
   a. Tomar antibióticos
   b. Usar cremas hidratantes
   c. Evitar el sol
   d. Hacer ejercicio regularmente

2. **¿Qué debe evitar el paciente para reducir los brotes de eczema?**
   a. Comer frutas
   b. Beber agua
   c. Usar jabones y detergentes fuertes
   d. Usar ropa de algodón

3. **¿Qué tipo de tratamiento médico menciona el dermatólogo?**
   a. Antihistamínicos
   b. Antibióticos
   c. Cremas con corticosteroides
   d. Inyecciones de vitaminas

Dialogue 48: Eczema Management - Manejo del eczema

Dermatologist: Good morning. Let's take care of your skin and talk about managing your eczema.

Patient: Good morning, doctor. What can I do to control flare-ups?

Dermatologist: The most important thing is to keep your skin moisturized. Use special creams for sensitive skin.

Patient: Is there anything I should avoid?

Dermatologist: Avoid strong soaps and detergents that irritate. And remember, don't scratch to prevent further damage to your skin.

Patient: Does diet influence eczema?

Dermatologist: Sometimes, certain foods can make it worse. I'll help you identify them with a food diary.

Patient: Are there medical treatments for eczema?

Dermatologist: Yes, there are corticosteroid creams that relieve inflammation. I'll show you how to use them correctly.

Comprehension Questions

1. **What is the main approach to managing eczema according to the dermatologist?**
   a. Taking antibiotics
   b. Using moisturizing creams
   c. Avoiding the sun
   d. Regular exercise

2. **What should the patient avoid to reduce eczema flare-ups?**
   a. Eating fruits
   b. Drinking water
   c. Using harsh soaps and detergents
   d. Wearing cotton clothes

3. **What type of medical treatment does the dermatologist mention?**
   a. Antihistamines
   b. Antibiotics
   c. Corticosteroid creams
   d. Vitamin injections

Answers

1. **b)** Usar cremas hidratantes - Using moisturizing creams
2. **c)** Usar jabones y detergentes fuertes - Using harsh soaps and detergents
3. **a)** Antihistamínicos - Antihistamines

Tratamiento del acné - Acne Treatment

Dermatólogo: Buenos días. Vamos a hablar sobre el tratamiento adecuado para tu acné.

Paciente: Buenos días. ¿Qué puedo hacer para mejorar mi piel?

Dermatólogo: Primero, es importante limpiar la piel suavemente con un limpiador adecuado para el acné.

Paciente: ¿Debo usar algún tipo de crema o medicamento?

Dermatólogo: Sí, te prescribiré una crema con retinoides que ayuda a prevenir los brotes.

Paciente: ¿Hay algo que debería evitar en mi dieta o estilo de vida?

Dermatólogo: Algunas personas notan que ciertos alimentos como los lácteos o alimentos grasosos pueden empeorar el acné. Mantén una dieta equilibrada.

Paciente: ¿Y el maquillaje tiene algo que ver?

Dermatólogo: Utiliza maquillaje no comedogénico para evitar tapar los poros.

Paciente: ¿Cuánto tiempo tardaré en ver resultados?

Dermatólogo: El tratamiento del acné puede tardar varias semanas para mostrar mejoría. Es importante ser constante y paciente.

Preguntas de comprensión

1. **¿Qué recomienda el dermatólogo para la limpieza de la piel?**
   a. Jabones fuertes
   b. Limpiador suave para el acné
   c. No lavar la cara
   d. Sólo agua

2. **¿Qué tipo de crema prescribirá el dermatólogo?**
   a. Crema hidratante
   b. Crema con antibióticos
   c. Crema con retinoides
   d. Crema bronceadora

3. **¿Qué consejo da el dermatólogo sobre el uso de maquillaje?**
   a. No usar maquillaje
   b. Usar maquillaje no comedogénico
   c. Usar sólo maquillaje natural
   d. Aplicar mucho maquillaje

Dialogue 49:

Acne Treatment - Tratamiento del acné

Dermatologist: Good morning. Let's talk about the appropriate treatment for your acne.

Patient: Good morning. What can I do to improve my skin?

Dermatologist: First, it's important to gently cleanse your skin with a cleanser suitable for acne.

Patient: Should I use any specific cream or medication?

Dermatologist: Yes, I'll prescribe a cream with retinoids that helps to prevent breakouts.

Patient: Is there anything I should avoid in my diet or lifestyle?

Dermatologist: Some people find that certain foods, like dairy or fatty foods, can worsen acne. Keep a balanced diet.

Patient: What about makeup?

Dermatologist: Use non-comedogenic makeup to avoid clogging pores.

Patient: How long will it take to see results?

Dermatologist: Acne treatment can take several weeks to show improvement. It's important to be consistent and patient.

Comprehension Questions

1. **What does the dermatologist recommend for skin cleansing?**
   a. Strong soaps
   b. Gentle acne cleanser
   c. Not washing the face
   d. Only water

2. **What type of cream will the dermatologist prescribe?**
   a. Moisturizing cream
   b. Antibiotic cream
   c. Retinoid cream
   d. Tanning cream

3. **What advice does the dermatologist give about using makeup?**
   a. Do not use makeup
   b. Use non-comedogenic makeup
   c. Use only natural makeup
   d. Apply a lot of makeup

Answers

1. **b)** Limpiador suave para el acné - Gentle acne cleanser
2. **c)** Crema con retinoides - Retinoid cream
3. **b)** Usar maquillaje no comedogénico - Use non-comedogenic makeup

Alergia en la piel - Skin Allergy

Dermatólogo: Buenos días. Hoy hablaremos de tu alergia en la piel y cómo manejarla.

Paciente: Buenos días. ¿Qué debo hacer para aliviar los síntomas?

Dermatólogo: Es fundamental identificar y evitar los alérgenos que desencadenan tu reacción.

Paciente: ¿Cómo puedo saber qué me causa la alergia?

Dermatólogo: Podemos hacer pruebas de alergias para identificar los alérgenos específicos.

Paciente: ¿Hay algún tratamiento que pueda usar para la comezón?

Dermatólogo: Sí, te recomendaré cremas con corticosteroides y antihistamínicos orales para aliviar el picor y la inflamación.

Paciente: ¿Debo cambiar algo en mi rutina de cuidado de la piel?

Dermatólogo: Sí, usa productos hipoalergénicos y evita aquellos con fragancias o conservantes que puedan irritar tu piel.

Paciente: ¿Estas alergias pueden desaparecer con el tiempo?

Dermatólogo: Algunas alergias cutáneas pueden disminuir o desaparecer, pero es importante continuar evitando los alérgenos conocidos.

Preguntas de comprensión

1. **¿Qué es esencial para manejar la alergia en la piel según el dermatólogo?**
   a. Usar siempre protector solar
   b. Identificar y evitar los alérgenos
   c. Bañarse con agua caliente
   d. Tomar antibióticos

2. **¿Qué tipo de pruebas puede sugerir el dermatólogo?**
   a. Pruebas de glucosa en sangre
   b. Pruebas de la presión arterial
   c. Pruebas de alergias
   d. Biopsias de la piel

3. **¿Qué tipo de productos para la piel recomienda el dermatólogo?**
   a. Productos con alcohol
   b. Productos hipoalergénicos
   c. Productos con fragancias fuertes
   d. Productos exfoliantes

Dialogue 50:
Skin Allergy - Alergia en la piel

Dermatologist: Good morning. Today we will address your skin allergy and how to manage it.

Patient: Good morning. What should I do to relieve the symptoms?

Dermatologist: It's crucial to identify and avoid the allergens that trigger your reaction.

Patient: How can I find out what causes my allergy?

Dermatologist: We can perform allergy tests to identify specific allergens.

Patient: Is there any treatment I can use for the itching?

Dermatologist: Yes, I will recommend corticosteroid creams and oral antihistamines to relieve itching and inflammation.

Patient: Should I change anything in my skincare routine?

Dermatologist: Yes, use hypoallergenic products and avoid those with fragrances or preservatives that may irritate your skin.

Patient: Can these allergies go away over time?

Dermatologist: Some skin allergies may diminish or disappear, but it's important to continue avoiding known allergens.

Comprehension Questions

1. **What is essential for managing skin allergy according to the dermatologist?**
   a. Always use sunscreen
   b. Identify and avoid allergens
   c. Bathe with hot water
   d. Take antibiotics

2. **What type of tests might the dermatologist suggest?**
   a. Blood sugar tests
   b. Blood pressure tests
   c. Allergy tests
   d. Skin biopsies

3. **What kind of skin care products does the dermatologist recommend?**
   a. Products with alcohol
   b. Hypoallergenic products
   c. Products with strong fragrances
   d. Exfoliating products

Answers

1. **b)** Identificar y evitar los alérgenos - Identify and avoid allergens
2. **c)** Pruebas de alergias - Allergy tests
3. **b)** Productos hipoalergénicos - Hypoallergenic products

Key Preventive Care Concepts

Vaccinations (Vacunaciones)

Diálogo:

Doctor: "Es esencial mantener sus vacunas al día para prevenir enfermedades graves. Las vacunas ayudan a su sistema inmunológico a luchar contra infecciones".

Paciente: «¿Qué vacunas necesito?»

Doctor: "Depende de su edad y condiciones de salud. Por ejemplo, la vacuna contra la gripe se recomienda anualmente".

Dialogue:

Doctor: "It's essential to keep your vaccinations up to date to prevent serious diseases. Vaccines help your immune system fight off infections."

Patient: "Which vaccines do I need?"

Doctor: "It depends on your age and health conditions. For example, the flu vaccine is recommended annually."

Comprehension Check

1. "Para prevenir la gripe, se recomienda la vacuna _____".

   Options: a) anualmente   b) mensualmente   c) semanalmente

   _____

2. "Las vacunas ayudan a su sistema inmunológico a _____ contra infecciones."

   Options: a) olvidar   b) descansar   c) luchar

   _____

3. ¿Por qué son importantes las vacunaciones según el doctor?

   _____

1. **a) anualmente (annually)**

   "Para prevenir la gripe, se recomienda la vacuna **(anualmente)**".

2. **c) luchar (fight)**

   "Las vacunas ayudan a su sistema inmunológico a **(luchar)** contra infecciones".

3. **¿Por qué son importantes las vacunaciones según el doctor?**

   Why are vaccinations important according to the doctor?

   - Las vacunaciones son importantes porque ayudan a prevenir enfermedades graves y a proteger el sistema inmunológico.
   - Vaccinations are important because they help prevent serious diseases and protect the immune system.

   _____

   _____

   _____

   _____

Regular Health Check-Ups (Revisiones médicas regulares)

The necessity of routine medical examinations for early detection of health issues.

Diálogo:

Doctor: "Es fundamental realizar revisiones médicas regulares para la detección temprana de problemas de salud. Estos exámenes nos ayudan a identificar cualquier cambio en su estado de salud".

Paciente: «¿Con qué frecuencia debo hacerme una revisión?"

Doctor: "Recomendamos que sea anual, pero podría variar según su edad y condiciones de salud".

Dialogue:

Doctor: "Regular health check-ups are crucial for early detection of health issues. These exams help us identify any changes in your health status."

Patient: "How often should I get a check-up?"

Doctor: "We recommend an annual check-up, but it may vary depending on your age and medical conditions."

Comprehension Check

1. "Se recomienda una revisión _____ para la detección temprana de problemas de salud".

    Options: a) semanal   b) mensual   c) anual

    _____

2. "Las revisiones médicas regulares ayudan a identificar _____ en su estado de salud".

    Options: a) cambios   b) errores   c) olvidos

    _____

3. ¿Con qué frecuencia se recomienda hacerse una revisión según el doctor?

    _____

Answers – Regular Health Check-Ups (Revisiones médicas regulares)

1. **c) anual (annual)**

   "Se recomienda una revisión **(anual)** para la detección temprana de problemas de salud".

2. **a) cambios (changes)**

   "Los chequeos de salud regulares ayudan a identificar **(cambios)** en su estado de salud".

3. **¿Con qué frecuencia se recomienda hacerse una revisiónsegún el doctor?**

   How often does the doctor recommend getting a check-up?

   - El doctor recomienda una revisión anual, pero puede variar según la edad y condiciones de salud.
   - The doctor recommends an annual check-up, but it may vary depending on age and medical conditions

   _____

   _____

   _____

   _____

Healthy Diet (Dieta saludable)

Emphasizing balanced nutrition for overall health.

Diálogo:

Nutricionista: "Una dieta saludable es clave para mantener una buena salud. Incluya una variedad de frutas, verduras, proteínas magras y granos enteros en su dieta diaria".

Paciente: «¿Debo evitar ciertos alimentos?»

Nutricionista: "Limite el consumo de alimentos procesados, azúcares añadidos y grasas saturadas para mejorar su bienestar general".

Dialogue:

Nutritionist: "A healthy diet is key to maintaining good health. Include a variety of fruits, vegetables, lean proteins, and whole grains in your daily diet."

Patient: "Should I avoid certain foods?"

Nutritionist: "Limit the intake of processed foods, added sugars, and saturated fats to improve your overall well-being."

Comprehension Check

1. "Una dieta saludable incluye una variedad de _____".

   Options: a) dulces   b) frutas y verduras   c) bebidas gaseosas

   _____

2. "Para mejorar el bienestar general, se debe limitar el consumo de alimentos _____".

   Options: a) frescos   b) procesados   c) caseros

   _____

3. ¿Qué alimentos recomienda limitar el nutricionista para una dieta saludable?

   _____

Answers – Healthy Diet (Dieta saludable)

1. **b) frutas y verduras (fruits and vegetables)**

    "Una dieta saludable incluye una variedad de **(frutas y verduras)**".

2. **b) procesados (processed)**

    "Para mejorar el bienestar general, se debe limitar el consumo de alimentos **(procesados)**".

3. **¿Qué alimentos recomienda limitar el nutricionista para una dieta saludable?**

    What foods does the nutritionist recommend limiting for a healthy diet?

    - El nutricionista recomienda limitar el consumo de alimentos procesados, azúcares añadidos y grasas saturadas.

    - The nutritionist recommends limiting the intake of processed foods, added sugars, and saturated fats.

    _____

    _____

    _____

    _____

Physical Activity (Actividad física):

The role of regular exercise in maintaining good health.

Diálogo:

Doctor: "Es importante incorporar actividad física en su rutina diaria para mantenerse saludable. El ejercicio regular fortalece el corazón y mejora la circulación".

Paciente: «¿Qué tipo de ejercicio debería hacer?»

Doctor: "Caminar, nadar, o andar en bicicleta son buenas opciones. Lo importante es elegir una actividad que disfrute y ser constante".

Dialogue:

Doctor: "It's important to incorporate physical activity into your daily routine to stay healthy. Regular exercise strengthens the heart and improves circulation."

Patient: "What type of exercise should I do?"

Doctor: "Walking, swimming, or cycling are good options. The key is to choose an activity you enjoy and be consistent with it."

Comprehension Check

1. "Para mantener un corazón saludable, es importante hacer ejercicio
   _____".

   Options: a) ocasionalmente b) raramente   c) regularmente

   _____

2. "_____ son buenas opciones para el ejercicio, según el doctor".

   Options: a) Dormir y descansar b) Caminar y nadar c) Comer y beber

   _____

3. ¿Cuál es el papel del ejercicio físico en la salud según el doctor?

   _____

1. **c) regularmente (regularly)**

   "Para mantener un corazón saludable, es importante hacer ejercicio **(regularmente)**".

2. **b) Caminar y nadar (Walking and swimming)**

   "**(Caminar y nadar)** son buenas opciones para el ejercicio, según el doctor".

3. **¿Cuál es el papel del ejercicio físico en la salud según el doctor?**

   What is the role of physical exercise in health according to the doctor?

   - El ejercicio físico fortalece el corazón y mejora la circulación.
   - Physical activity strengthens the heart and improves circulation.

   _____

   _____

   _____

   _____

Stress Management (Manejo del estrés)

Techniques and importance of managing stress for mental well-being.

Diálogo:

Doctor: "Manejar el estrés es crucial para su salud mental. Técnicas como la meditación y la respiración profunda pueden ser muy efectivas".

Paciente: «¿Qué más puedo hacer para reducir el estrés?»

Doctor: "Es importante también hacer ejercicio regularmente y mantener una rutina de sueño saludable. Dése tiempo para actividades relajantes".

Dialogue:

Doctor: "Managing stress is crucial for your mental health. Techniques like meditation and deep breathing can be very effective."

Patient: "What else can I do to reduce stress?"

Doctor: "Regular exercise and maintaining a healthy sleep routine are also important. Make time for relaxing activities."

Comprehension Check

1. "La meditación y la _____ profunda son técnicas efectivas para el manejo del estrés".

   Options: a) caminata   b) alimentación   c) respiración

   _____

2. "Para reducir el estrés, es importante mantener una rutina de _____ saludable".

   Options: a) trabajo   b) sueño   c) alimentación

   _____

3. ¿Por qué es importante manejar el estrés según el doctor?

   _____

Answers – Stress Management (Manejo del estrés)

1. **c) respiración (breathing)**

   "La meditación y la **(respiración)** profunda son técnicas efectivas para el manejo del estrés".

2. **b) sueño (sleep)**

   "Para reducir el estrés, es importante mantener una rutina de **(sueño)** saludable".

3. **¿Por qué es importante manejar el estrés?**

   Why is it important to manage stress?

   - Manejar el estrés es crucial para la salud mental.
   - Managing stress is crucial for mental health.

   _____

   _____

   _____

   _____

Avoiding Tobacco and Alcohol (Prevención del consumo de tabaco y alcohol)

Discussing the health risks associated with smoking and excessive alcohol consumption.

Diálogo:

Doctor: "Evitar el tabaco y el consumo excesivo de alcohol es vital para su salud. Ambos pueden causar enfermedades graves".

Paciente: «¿Cómo puedo reducir el consumo de alcohol?»

Doctor: "Es importante fijar límites y buscar apoyo. También evite situaciones donde se sienta tentado a beber".

Dialogue:

Doctor: "Avoiding tobacco and excessive alcohol use is vital for your health. Both can cause serious diseases."

Patient: "How can I reduce alcohol consumption?"

Doctor: "Setting limits and seeking support are important steps. Also, avoid situations where you feel tempted to drink."

Comprehension Check

1. "Evitar el _____ es vital para prevenir enfermedades graves".

   Options: a) ejercicio   b) tabaco   c) azúcar

   _____

2. "Para reducir el consumo de alcohol, es importante fijar _____ y buscar apoyo".

   Options: a) límites   b) amigos   c) recetas

   _____

3. ¿Cuál es el riesgo de fumar y beber en exceso según el doctor?

   _____

Answers – Avoiding Tobacco and Alcohol
(Prevención del consumo de tabaco y alcohol)

1. **b) tabaco (tobacco)**
   "Evitar el **(tabaco)** es vital para prevenir enfermedades graves".

2. **b) límites (limits)**
   "Para reducir el consumo de alcohol, es importante fijar **(límites)** y buscar apoyo".

3. **¿Cuál es el riesgo de fumar y beber en exceso según el doctor?**
   What is the risk of smoking and excessive drinking according to the doctor?

   - Fumar y beber en exceso pueden causar enfermedades graves.
   - Smoking and excessive drinking can cause serious diseases.

   _____

   _____

   _____

   _____

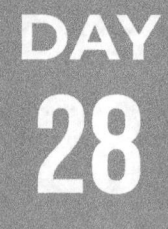
Screenings for Chronic Diseases
(Detección de enfermedades crónicas)

The importance of screenings for conditions like diabetes, hypertension, and high cholesterol.

Diálogo:

Doctor: "Realizar exámenes regulares es clave para la detección temprana de enfermedades crónicas como la diabetes y la hipertensión".

Paciente: «¿Con qué frecuencia debo hacerme estos exámenes?»

Doctor: "Depende de factores como su edad e historial médico. Generalmente se recomiendan una vez al año".

Dialogue:

Doctor: "Regular screenings are key to early detection of chronic diseases like diabetes and hypertension."

Patient: "How often should I get these screenings?"

Doctor: "It depends on factors like your age and medical history. Generally, once a year is advisable."

Comprehension Check

1. "Realizar exámenes regulares es clave para detectar pronto enfermedades como la _____ y la hipertensión".

   Options: a) diabetes   b) osteoporosis   c) anemia

   _____

2. "Según su edad e historial médico, se recomienda hacer exámenes al menos una vez al _____".

   Options: a) mes   b) año   c) día

   _____

3. ¿Cuál es la importancia de los exámenes regulares según el doctor?

   _____

Answers – Screenings for Chronic Diseases
(Detección de enfermedades crónicas)

1. **a) diabetes (diabetes)**
   "Realizar exámenes regulares es clave para detectar pronto enfermedades como la **(diabetes)** y la hipertensión".

2. **b) año (year)**
   "Según su edad e historial médico, se recomienda hacer exámenes al menos una vez al **(año)**".

3. **¿Cuál es la importancia de los exámenes regulares según el doctor?**
   What is the importance of regular examinations according to the doctor?

   - Los exámenes regulares son clave para la detección temprana de enfermedades crónicas.
   - Regular screenings are key to early detection of chronic diseases.

   _____

   _____

   _____

   _____

Mental Health Awareness (Conciencia sobre la salud mental)

Recognizing and addressing mental health concerns.

Diálogo:

Doctor: "Hablar sobre la salud mental es tan importante como cuidar de la salud física. ¿Cómo se ha sentido últimamente?"

Paciente: "He estado un poco ansioso y tengo problemas para dormir".

Doctor: "Vamos a hablar sobre esto y ver cuáles recursos y tratamientos podrían ayudarle".

Dialogue:

Doctor: "Discussing mental health is as important as taking care of physical health. How have you been feeling lately?"

Patient: "I've been a bit anxious and having trouble sleeping."

Doctor: "Let's talk about this and see what support and treatments might help you."

Comprehension Check

1. "Hablar sobre la salud mental es tan importante como cuidar de la _____ física".

   Options: a) salud   b) alimentación   c) actividad

   _____

2. "El paciente menciona sentirse _____ y tener problemas para dormir".

   Options: a) feliz   b) ansioso   c) energético

   _____

3. ¿Cuál es la importancia de hablar sobre la salud mental según el doctor?

   _____

Answers – Mental Health Awareness (Conciencia sobre la salud mental)

1. **a) salud (health)**

   "Hablar sobre la salud mental es tan importante como cuidar de la **(salud)** física».

2. **b) ansioso (anxious)**

   "El paciente menciona sentirse **(ansioso)** y tener problemas para dormir".

3. **¿Cuál es la importancia de hablar sobre la salud mental según el doctor?**

   What is the importance of talking about mental health according to the doctor?

   - Hablar sobre la salud mental es tan importante como cuidar de la salud física.
   - (Discussing mental health is as important as taking care of physical health.)

   _____

   _____

   _____

   _____

Sleep Hygiene (Higiene del sueño)

The importance of quality sleep and its impact on health.

Diálogo:

Doctor: "Un sueño de calidad es fundamental para su salud general. ¿Cómo son sus hábitos de sueño?"

Paciente: "A menudo me cuesta dormir y me despierto cansado".

Doctor: "Veamos estrategias para mejorar su higiene del sueño, como establecer una rutina y evitar pantallas antes de dormir".

Dialogue:

Doctor: "Quality sleep is essential for your overall health. How are your sleeping habits?"

Patient: "I often have trouble sleeping and wake up feeling tired."

Doctor: "Let's explore strategies to improve your sleep hygiene, like establishing a routine and avoiding screens before bed."

Comprehension Check

1. "Un sueño de _____ es fundamental para su salud general".

   Options: a) interrumpido b) calidad c) excesivo

   _____

2. "El paciente tiene problemas para _____ y se despierta cansado".

   Options: a) comer b) dormir c) correr

   _____

3. ¿Cuál es la importancia de una buena higiene del sueño según el doctor?

   _____

Answers – Sleep Hygiene (Higiene del sueño)

1. **b) calidad (quality)**

    "Un sueño de **(calidad)** es fundamental para su salud general".

2. **b) dormir (sleep)**

    "El paciente tiene problemas para **(dormir)** y se despierta cansado**".**

3. **¿Cuál es la importancia de una buena higiene del sueño según el doctor?**

    What is the importance of good sleep hygiene according to the doctor?

    - Una buena higiene del sueño es fundamental para la salud general.
    - Good sleep hygiene is essential for overall health.

    _____

    _____

    _____

Sun Protection (Protección solar)

Preventing skin damage and skin cancer through sun safety.

Diálogo:

Doctor: "La protección solar es clave para prevenir daños en la piel y el cáncer de piel. Recomiendo usar protector solar diariamente".

Paciente: «¿Qué factor de protección solar debo usar?»

Doctor: "Un SPF de al menos 30 es ideal, especialmente si va a estar al aire libre durante mucho tiempo".

Dialogue:

Doctor: "Sun protection is key to preventing skin damage and skin cancer. I recommend using sunscreen daily."

Patient: "What SPF should I use?"

Doctor: "An SPF of at least 30 is ideal, especially if you're going to be outdoors for an extended period."

Comprehension Check

1. "La protección solar es clave para prevenir _____ en la piel".

   Options: a) humedad   b) bronceado   c) daños

   _____

2. "Un SPF de al menos _____ es ideal para la protección solar".

   Options: a) 10   b) 30   c) 50

   _____

3. ¿Cuál es la importancia de la protección solar según el doctor?

   _____

Answers – Sun Protection (Protección solar)

1. **c) daños (damage)**
    "La protección solar es clave para prevenir **(daños)** en la piel".

2. **b) 30 (thirty)**
    "Un SPF de al menos **(30)** es ideal para la protección solar".

3. **¿Cuál es la importancia de la protección solar según el doctor?**
    What is the importance of sun protection according to the doctor?

    - La protección solar es fundamental para prevenir daños en la piel y el cáncer de piel.
    - Sun protection is crucial for preventing skin damage and skin cancer.

    _____

    _____

    _____

    _____

BUILDING LANGUAGE SKILLS

Advanced Grammar Concepts

Step into the linguist's lab coat as we tackle 'Advanced Grammar Concepts' in the medical Spanish realm! The 'Conditional Mood' is your go-to for discussing patient prognoses and treatment plans with a twist of 'what could happen.' Then, with the 'Subjunctive Mood,' you'll learn to articulate hopes and recommendations for your patients, adding a layer of compassion to your consults. It's all about giving you the tools to communicate complex medical ideas with ease and a dash of personality!

The Conditional Mood

The conditional mood in Spanish is used to express actions that would happen under certain conditions. It's often used to talk about hypothetical situations, probabilities, and to give polite suggestions or advice. In medical scenarios, it's particularly useful when discussing potential treatment plans, outcomes, or advising patients on health management.

Short Story

Dr. Fernandez is discussing a treatment plan with Mr. Lopez, who has recently been diagnosed with diabetes. Mr. Lopez is concerned about the changes he needs to make in his lifestyle. Dr. Fernandez explains that if Mr. Lopez follows a balanced diet and exercises regularly, he would likely see an improvement in his health. She also mentions that, ideally, he should monitor his blood sugar levels daily.

Now let's look at how to use the conditional mood.

1. **Discussing Potential Treatments**

   Original Verb: mejorar (to improve)

   Conditional: mejoraría (would improve)

   - If you followed this treatment, your condition **would improve**.
   - Si usted siguiera este tratamiento, su condición **mejoraría**.

   Trigger: Si usted siguiera (If you followed)

   _____

   _____

2. **Advising on Lifestyle Changes**

   Original Verb: controlar (to control)

   Subjunctive: controlaría (would control)

   - Exercising regularly **would control** your blood sugar levels.
   - Hacer ejercicio regularmente **controlaría** sus niveles de azúcar en sangre.

   _____

   _____

3. **Discussing Probabilities**

   Original Verb: necesitar (to need)

   Conditional: necesitaría (would need)

   - You **would need** to check your blood sugar daily.
   - Usted **necesitaría** revisar su azúcar en sangre diariamente.

   _____

   _____

4. **Giving Polite Suggestions**

   Original Verb: tomar (to take)

   Subjunctive: tomaría (would take)

   - You **would take** this medication twice a day.
   - Usted **tomaría** este medicamento dos veces al día.

   _____

   _____

5. **Discussing Future Outcomes**

   Original Verb: ser (to be)

   Subjunctive: sería (would be)

   - It **would be** beneficial to join a support group for diabetes management.
   - **Sería** beneficioso unirse a un grupo de apoyo para el manejo de la diabetes.

   _____

   _____

Question 1:

- If you exercise regularly, your health <u>would improve</u>.
- Si haces ejercicio regularmente, tu salud _____.

   Options: a) mejoraría   b) mejora   c) mejorando

Question 2:

- For better sleep, you <u>would avoid</u> caffeine in the evening.
- Para dormir mejor, usted _____ la cafeína por la noche.

   Options: a) evitarías   b) evitaba   c) evitaría

Question 3:

- If I were in your place, I <u>would consult</u> a specialist.
- Si estuviera en tu lugar, yo _____ a un especialista.

   Options: a) consulto   b) consultaría   c) consultaba

Question 4:

- Taking this medicine <u>would reduce</u> the symptoms.
- Tomar esta medicina _____ los síntomas.

   Options: a) reduciría   b) reduce   c) reduciendo

Question 5:

- In your case, a diet change <u>would help</u> significantly.
- En tu caso, un cambio de dieta _____ significativamente.

   Options: a) ayudarías   b) ayudaría   c) ayuda

Answers

1. **a)** mejoraría
2. **c)** evitaría
3. **b)** consultaría
4. **a)** reduciría
5. **b)** ayudaría

A Short Story Using The Conditional Mood

In the following story, pay attention to the various instances where the conditional mood is being used. Write down as many as you can or if you're following along with the companion document, fill in the blanks provided.

Read the story below and underline each time the conditional mood is used. Then fill in the blanks with your findings.

El doctor García habla con su paciente, Ana.

"Si tomara este medicamento, podría mejorar su diabetes", dice el doctor.

"Pero debería evitar los alimentos con mucha azúcar y grasas. Si hiciera ejercicio regularmente, su salud mejoraría notablemente.

También, si redujera el estrés en su vida, se sentiría más relajada y saludable.

Este tratamiento podría ser efectivo, pero necesitaría su compromiso.

Si decidiera seguir estas recomendaciones, vería una gran diferencia en su salud".

1. _____

2. _____

3. _____

4. _____

5. _____

6. _____

7. _____

1. **podría mejorar** (could improve)
2. **debería evitar** (should avoid)
3. **mejoraría** (would improve)
4. **se sentiría** (would feel)
5. **podría ser** (could be)
6. **necesitaría** (would need)
7. **vería** (would see)

The Subjunctive Mood

The subjunctive mood in Spanish is used to express doubts, wishes, emotions, possibilities, and hypothetical situations. It's a way to describe things that are not certain to happen. In a medical context, the subjunctive mood can be particularly useful when giving advice, making recommendations, or discussing potential outcomes of a patient's condition. When one of these trigger words or phrases is used, the subjunctive conjugation of the verb is used.

Short Story

Maria, a worried mother, visits Dr. Lopez with her son, feeling unwell. She hopes for his quick recovery. Dr. Lopez recommends rest and hydration, but no antibiotics yet. Maria, still concerned, wonders about the vaccine's side effects. Dr. Lopez reassures her, emphasizing the need for close monitoring and promising prompt action if his condition worsens. Maria leaves, slightly relieved but still anxious.

Now let's look at how to use the subjunctive mood.

1. **Expressing a Wish**

    Original Verb: mejorar (to improve)

    Subjunctive: mejore (improves - subjunctive form)

    - The mother <u>hopes</u> her son **improves** soon.
    - La madre <u>espera que</u> su hijo **mejore** pronto

        Trigger: La madre <u>espera que</u> (The mother hopes that)

2. Giving a Recommendation

Original Verb: seguir (to follow)

Subjunctive: siga (follows - subjunctive form)

- The pediatrician <u>suggests</u> the child **follows** a balanced diet.
- El doctor <u>sugiere que</u> el niño **siga** una dieta balanceada.

   Trigger: El pediatra <u>sugiere que</u> (The pediatrician suggests that)

_____

_____

3. Discussing a Possibility

Original Verb: ser (to be)

Subjunctive: sea (is - subjunctive form)

- <u>It's possible that</u> the fever **is** a reaction to the vaccine.
- <u>Es posible que</u> la fiebre **sea** una reacción a la vacuna.

   Trigger: <u>Es posible que</u> (It's possible that)

_____

_____

4. Expressing Doubt or Uncertainty

Original Verb: necesitar (to need)

Subjunctive: necesite (needs - subjunctive form)

- The mother <u>doubts</u> her son **needs** antibiotics.
- La madre <u>duda que</u> su hijo **necesite** antibióticos.

   Trigger: La madre <u>duda que</u> (The mother doubts that)

_____

_____

5. Expressing a Desire

Original Verb: descansar (to rest)

Subjunctive: descanse (rests - subjunctive form)

- The mother <u>wants</u> her son to **<u>rest</u>** more during the illness.
- La madre <u>quiere que</u> su hijo **<u>descanse</u>** más durante la enfermedad.

  Trigger: La madre <u>quiere que</u> (The mother wants that)

Comprehension Check!

Question 1:

- It's important that the patient _____ a balanced diet to improve their health.
- Es importante que el paciente _____ una dieta equilibrada para mejorar su salud.

  Options: a) sigue   b) siga   c) seguía

Question 2:

- The doctor recommends that she _____ her medication regularly.
- El médico recomienda que ella _____ su medicamento regularmente.

  Options: a) toma   b) tome   c) tomaba

Question 3:

- I doubt that this treatment _____ effective for the patient.
- Dudo que este tratamiento _____ efectivo para el paciente.

  Options: a) sea   b) es   c) estaba

Question 4:

- It's possible that the patient _____ allergic to the medication.
- Es posible que el paciente _____ alérgico al medicamento.

  Options: a) es   b) era   c) sea

Question 5:

- I want my child to _____ more during his illness.
- Quiero que mi hijo _____ más durante su enfermedad.

Options: a) descansa   b) descansaba   c) descanse

Answers

1. **b)** siga
2. **b)** tome
3. **a)** sea
4. **c)** sea
5. **c)** descanse

A Short Story Using The Subjunctive Mood

In the following story, pay attention to the various instances where the subjunctive mood is being used.

Write them down as you hear them or if you're following along with the companion document, fill in the blanks provided.

Read the story below and underline each time the subjunctive mood is used. Then fill in the blanks with your findings.

La enfermera López aconseja a Carlos, quien acaba de tener una cirugía.

"Es importante que descanse bien después de la operación", le dice.

"Quiero que evite levantar objetos pesados y que tome sus medicamentos según lo recetado.

Es mejor que comunique si siente algún dolor fuerte o inusual.

Espero que siga todas estas instrucciones para una recuperación rápida.

Si nota alguna señal de infección como enrojecimiento o hinchazón, contacte inmediatamente al hospital.

Queremos que se recupere completamente y sin complicaciones".

1. _____

2. _____

3. _____

4. _____

5. _____

6. _____

7. _____

Answers

1. **descanse** bien (rest well)
2. **evite** levantar (avoid lifting)
3. **tome** sus medicamentos (take your medications)
4. **comunique** si siente (communicate if you feel)
5. **siga** las instrucciones (follow the instructions)
6. **nota** alguna señal (notice any sign)
7. **contacte** inmediatamente (contact immediately)
8. **se recupere** completamente (recover completely)

PATHWAY TO INTERMEDIATE LEARNING

Congratulations on reaching this extraordinary milestone in your Medical Spanish journey! From the modest start of grappling with basic phrases to now, marvel at your transformation! You're effortlessly navigating through intricate medical dialogues, a testament to your dedication and prowess.

As we check off the incredible milestone in your journey, let's celebrate not just your mastery of a language but the remarkable leap you've made. This adventure has done more than teach you Spanish; it has equipped you with the keys to forge genuine, heartfelt connections in the healthcare universe.

Journey Recap: A Transformation in Medical Spanish

- **Mastery in Grammar and Pronunciation:** You've moved beyond basic grammar to mastering nuances in pronunciation, crucial for building trust with Spanish-speaking patients.
- **Expanded Medical Vocabulary:** Your newfound vocabulary stretches across various medical fields, enhancing your ability to discuss symptoms, treatments, and patient care effectively.
- **Diverse Scenario Engagement:** From emergency situations to chronic care, you've practiced real-life medical dialogues, readying you for any patient conversation.
- **Excellence in Patient Education:** You've learned to simplify complex medical jargon, empowering your patients with knowledge and understanding.
- **Real-World Application:** Bringing Learning to Life

Now picture yourself in a pediatric consultation, easing a parent's worries with your fluent Spanish, or walking a patient through post-operative care, ensuring they understand every step. These aren't just scenarios; they're glimpses into your future interactions.

Self-Assessment and Growth

Challenge yourself with complex medical scenarios. How would you handle a heart disease discussion now? Engage in role-playing to simulate real-life consultations, and assess your growth in confidence and communication.

Strategies for Continuous Growth

- Diverse Learning Resources: Dive into Spanish medical literature, utilize language apps, and listen to medical podcasts. Engage with stories, discoveries, and expert interviews.
- Regular Practice and Cultural Immersion: Make Spanish a part of your daily routine and immerse yourself in Spanish-speaking cultures through travel or local events.
- Feedback and Adaptation: Seek constructive feedback from native speakers, embracing corrections as stepping stones to accuracy.

Embarking on the Intermediate Path

With a solid foundation, now venture into the realm of intermediate medical Spanish. This is where advanced grammar and specialized terminology become your tools for deeper connections. Embrace real-world practice by volunteering at health clinics and joining medical Spanish workshops – these aren't just practice sessions; they're pivotal experiences for building confidence and skill.

Building Bridges with Every Conversation

Mastering medical Spanish goes beyond acquiring a skill; it's about creating bridges of understanding and compassion with a broader patient community. Your journey forward is lined with opportunities to apply your skills, enhancing patient care and professional growth.

Stay the Course: The Path to Proficiency

Remain steadfast in your commitment. With each conversation, each day of practice, you're not just learning – you're transforming the way you connect with patients. Envision a future where your proficiency in medical Spanish brings confidence and clarity to your consultations, impacting both your career and the lives of those you care for.

Before long, you'll not only be recognized as a skilled healthcare professional but also as a pivotal figure in bridging the gap for Spanish-speaking patients, dismantling language barriers and pioneering new avenues in compassionate patient care.